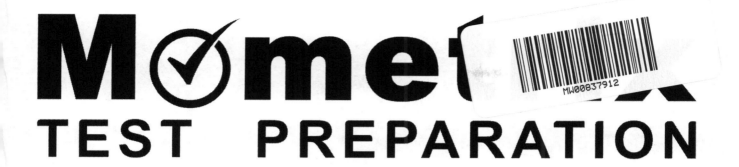

# NHA Phlebotomy

## Exam Secrets
## Study Guide

# DEAR FUTURE EXAM SUCCESS STORY

First of all, **THANK YOU** for purchasing Mometrix study materials!

Second, congratulations! You are one of the few determined test-takers who are committed to doing whatever it takes to excel on your exam. **You have come to the right place.** We developed these study materials with one goal in mind: to deliver you the information you need in a format that's concise and easy to use.

In addition to optimizing your guide for the content of the test, we've outlined our recommended steps for breaking down the preparation process into small, attainable goals so you can make sure you stay on track.

We've also analyzed the entire test-taking process, identifying the most common pitfalls and showing how you can overcome them and be ready for any curveball the test throws you.

Standardized testing is one of the biggest obstacles on your road to success, which only increases the importance of doing well in the high-pressure, high-stakes environment of test day. Your results on this test could have a significant impact on your future, and this guide provides the information and practical advice to help you achieve your full potential on test day.

### Your success is our success

**We would love to hear from you!** If you would like to share the story of your exam success or if you have any questions or comments in regard to our products, please contact us at **800-673-8175** or **support@mometrix.com**.

Thanks again for your business and we wish you continued success!

Sincerely,
The Mometrix Test Preparation Team

> **Need more help? Check out our flashcards at:**
> **http://MometrixFlashcards.com/Phlebotomy**

# TABLE OF CONTENTS

INTRODUCTION _____ 1

SECRET KEY #1 – PLAN BIG, STUDY SMALL _____ 2

SECRET KEY #2 – MAKE YOUR STUDYING COUNT _____ 3

SECRET KEY #3 – PRACTICE THE RIGHT WAY _____ 4

SECRET KEY #4 – PACE YOURSELF _____ 6

SECRET KEY #5 – HAVE A PLAN FOR GUESSING _____ 7

TEST-TAKING STRATEGIES _____ 10

SAFETY AND COMPLIANCE _____ 15

PATIENT PREPARATION _____ 24

ROUTINE BLOOD COLLECTIONS _____ 29

SPECIAL COLLECTIONS _____ 44

PROCESSING _____ 47

CORE KNOWLEDGE _____ 56

MEDICAL TERMINOLOGY _____ 71
    PREFIXES _____ 72
    SUFFIXES _____ 73
    WORD ROOTS _____ 75
    ACRONYMS AND ABBREVIATIONS _____ 79

NHA PRACTICE TEST _____ 84

ANSWER KEY AND EXPLANATIONS _____ 103

HOW TO OVERCOME TEST ANXIETY _____ 117
    CAUSES OF TEST ANXIETY _____ 117
    ELEMENTS OF TEST ANXIETY _____ 118
    EFFECTS OF TEST ANXIETY _____ 118
    PHYSICAL STEPS FOR BEATING TEST ANXIETY _____ 119
    MENTAL STEPS FOR BEATING TEST ANXIETY _____ 120
    STUDY STRATEGY _____ 121
    TEST TIPS _____ 123
    IMPORTANT QUALIFICATION _____ 124

THANK YOU _____ 125

ADDITIONAL BONUS MATERIAL _____ 126

# Introduction

**Thank you for purchasing this resource**! You have made the choice to prepare yourself for a test that could have a huge impact on your future, and this guide is designed to help you be fully ready for test day. Obviously, it's important to have a solid understanding of the test material, but you also need to be prepared for the unique environment and stressors of the test, so that you can perform to the best of your abilities.

For this purpose, the first section that appears in this guide is the **Secret Keys**. We've devoted countless hours to meticulously researching what works and what doesn't, and we've boiled down our findings to the five most impactful steps you can take to improve your performance on the test. We start at the beginning with study planning and move through the preparation process, all the way to the testing strategies that will help you get the most out of what you know when you're finally sitting in front of the test.

We recommend that you start preparing for your test as far in advance as possible. However, if you've bought this guide as a last-minute study resource and only have a few days before your test, we recommend that you skip over the first two Secret Keys since they address a long-term study plan.

If you struggle with **test anxiety**, we strongly encourage you to check out our recommendations for how you can overcome it. Test anxiety is a formidable foe, but it can be beaten, and we want to make sure you have the tools you need to defeat it.

# Secret Key #1 – Plan Big, Study Small

There's a lot riding on your performance. If you want to ace this test, you're going to need to keep your skills sharp and the material fresh in your mind. You need a plan that lets you review everything you need to know while still fitting in your schedule. We'll break this strategy down into three categories.

## Information Organization

Start with the information you already have: the official test outline. From this, you can make a complete list of all the concepts you need to cover before the test. Organize these concepts into groups that can be studied together, and create a list of any related vocabulary you need to learn so you can brush up on any difficult terms. You'll want to keep this vocabulary list handy once you actually start studying since you may need to add to it along the way.

## Time Management

Once you have your set of study concepts, decide how to spread them out over the time you have left before the test. Break your study plan into small, clear goals so you have a manageable task for each day and know exactly what you're doing. Then just focus on one small step at a time. When you manage your time this way, you don't need to spend hours at a time studying. Studying a small block of content for a short period each day helps you retain information better and avoid stressing over how much you have left to do. You can relax knowing that you have a plan to cover everything in time. In order for this strategy to be effective though, you have to start studying early and stick to your schedule. Avoid the exhaustion and futility that comes from last-minute cramming!

## Study Environment

The environment you study in has a big impact on your learning. Studying in a coffee shop, while probably more enjoyable, is not likely to be as fruitful as studying in a quiet room. It's important to keep distractions to a minimum. You're only planning to study for a short block of time, so make the most of it. Don't pause to check your phone or get up to find a snack. It's also important to **avoid multitasking**. Research has consistently shown that multitasking will make your studying dramatically less effective. Your study area should also be comfortable and well-lit so you don't have the distraction of straining your eyes or sitting on an uncomfortable chair.

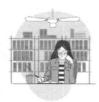 The time of day you study is also important. You want to be rested and alert. Don't wait until just before bedtime. Study when you'll be most likely to comprehend and remember. Even better, if you know what time of day your test will be, set that time aside for study. That way your brain will be used to working on that subject at that specific time and you'll have a better chance of recalling information.

Finally, it can be helpful to team up with others who are studying for the same test. Your actual studying should be done in as isolated an environment as possible, but the work of organizing the information and setting up the study plan can be divided up. In between study sessions, you can discuss with your teammates the concepts that you're all studying and quiz each other on the details. Just be sure that your teammates are as serious about the test as you are. If you find that your study time is being replaced with social time, you might need to find a new team.

2

# Secret Key #2 – Make Your Studying Count

You're devoting a lot of time and effort to preparing for this test, so you want to be absolutely certain it will pay off. This means doing more than just reading the content and hoping you can remember it on test day. It's important to make every minute of study count. There are two main areas you can focus on to make your studying count.

## Retention

It doesn't matter how much time you study if you can't remember the material. You need to make sure you are retaining the concepts. To check your retention of the information you're learning, try recalling it at later times with minimal prompting. Try carrying around flashcards and glance at one or two from time to time or ask a friend who's also studying for the test to quiz you.

To enhance your retention, look for ways to put the information into practice so that you can apply it rather than simply recalling it. If you're using the information in practical ways, it will be much easier to remember. Similarly, it helps to solidify a concept in your mind if you're not only reading it to yourself but also explaining it to someone else. Ask a friend to let you teach them about a concept you're a little shaky on (or speak aloud to an imaginary audience if necessary). As you try to summarize, define, give examples, and answer your friend's questions, you'll understand the concepts better and they will stay with you longer. Finally, step back for a big picture view and ask yourself how each piece of information fits with the whole subject. When you link the different concepts together and see them working together as a whole, it's easier to remember the individual components.

Finally, practice showing your work on any multi-step problems, even if you're just studying. Writing out each step you take to solve a problem will help solidify the process in your mind, and you'll be more likely to remember it during the test.

## Modality

*Modality* simply refers to the means or method by which you study. Choosing a study modality that fits your own individual learning style is crucial. No two people learn best in exactly the same way, so it's important to know your strengths and use them to your advantage.

For example, if you learn best by visualization, focus on visualizing a concept in your mind and draw an image or a diagram. Try color-coding your notes, illustrating them, or creating symbols that will trigger your mind to recall a learned concept. If you learn best by hearing or discussing information, find a study partner who learns the same way or read aloud to yourself. Think about how to put the information in your own words. Imagine that you are giving a lecture on the topic and record yourself so you can listen to it later.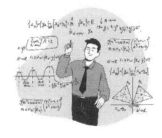

For any learning style, flashcards can be helpful. Organize the information so you can take advantage of spare moments to review. Underline key words or phrases. Use different colors for different categories. Mnemonic devices (such as creating a short list in which every item starts with the same letter) can also help with retention. Find what works best for you and use it to store the information in your mind most effectively and easily.

# Secret Key #3 – Practice the Right Way

Your success on test day depends not only on how many hours you put into preparing, but also on whether you prepared the right way. It's good to check along the way to see if your studying is paying off. One of the most effective ways to do this is by taking practice tests to evaluate your progress. Practice tests are useful because they show exactly where you need to improve. Every time you take a practice test, pay special attention to these three groups of questions:

- The questions you got wrong
- The questions you had to guess on, even if you guessed right
- The questions you found difficult or slow to work through

This will show you exactly what your weak areas are, and where you need to devote more study time. Ask yourself why each of these questions gave you trouble. Was it because you didn't understand the material? Was it because you didn't remember the vocabulary? Do you need more repetitions on this type of question to build speed and confidence? Dig into those questions and figure out how you can strengthen your weak areas as you go back to review the material.

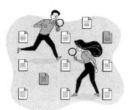 Additionally, many practice tests have a section explaining the answer choices. It can be tempting to read the explanation and think that you now have a good understanding of the concept. However, an explanation likely only covers part of the question's broader context. Even if the explanation makes perfect sense, **go back and investigate** every concept related to the question until you're positive you have a thorough understanding.

As you go along, keep in mind that the practice test is just that: practice. Memorizing these questions and answers will not be very helpful on the actual test because it is unlikely to have any of the same exact questions. If you only know the right answers to the sample questions, you won't be prepared for the real thing. **Study the concepts** until you understand them fully, and then you'll be able to answer any question that shows up on the test.

It's important to wait on the practice tests until you're ready. If you take a test on your first day of study, you may be overwhelmed by the amount of material covered and how much you need to learn. Work up to it gradually.

On test day, you'll need to be prepared for answering questions, managing your time, and using the test-taking strategies you've learned. It's a lot to balance, like a mental marathon that will have a big impact on your future. Like training for a marathon, you'll need to start slowly and work your way up. When test day arrives, you'll be ready.

Start with the strategies you've read in the first two Secret Keys—plan your course and study in the way that works best for you. If you have time, consider using multiple study resources to get different approaches to the same concepts. It can be helpful to see difficult concepts from more than one angle. Then find a good source for practice tests. Many times, the test website will suggest potential study resources or provide sample tests.

# Practice Test Strategy

If you're able to find at least three practice tests, we recommend this strategy:

## UNTIMED AND OPEN-BOOK PRACTICE

Take the first test with no time constraints and with your notes and study guide handy. Take your time and focus on applying the strategies you've learned.

## TIMED AND OPEN-BOOK PRACTICE

Take the second practice test open-book as well, but set a timer and practice pacing yourself to finish in time.

## TIMED AND CLOSED-BOOK PRACTICE

Take any other practice tests as if it were test day. Set a timer and put away your study materials. Sit at a table or desk in a quiet room, imagine yourself at the testing center, and answer questions as quickly and accurately as possible.

Keep repeating timed and closed-book tests on a regular basis until you run out of practice tests or it's time for the actual test. Your mind will be ready for the schedule and stress of test day, and you'll be able to focus on recalling the material you've learned.

# Secret Key #4 – Pace Yourself

Once you're fully prepared for the material on the test, your biggest challenge on test day will be managing your time. Just knowing that the clock is ticking can make you panic even if you have plenty of time left. Work on pacing yourself so you can build confidence against the time constraints of the exam. Pacing is a difficult skill to master, especially in a high-pressure environment, so **practice is vital**.

Set time expectations for your pace based on how much time is available. For example, if a section has 60 questions and the time limit is 30 minutes, you know you have to average 30 seconds or less per question in order to answer them all. Although 30 seconds is the hard limit, set 25 seconds per question as your goal, so you reserve extra time to spend on harder questions. When you budget extra time for the harder questions, you no longer have any reason to stress when those questions take longer to answer.

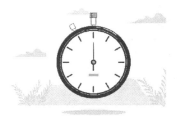

Don't let this time expectation distract you from working through the test at a calm, steady pace, but keep it in mind so you don't spend too much time on any one question. Recognize that taking extra time on one question you don't understand may keep you from answering two that you do understand later in the test. If your time limit for a question is up and you're still not sure of the answer, mark it and move on, and come back to it later if the time and the test format allow. If the testing format doesn't allow you to return to earlier questions, just make an educated guess; then put it out of your mind and move on.

On the easier questions, be careful not to rush. It may seem wise to hurry through them so you have more time for the challenging ones, but it's not worth missing one if you know the concept and just didn't take the time to read the question fully. Work efficiently but make sure you understand the question and have looked at all of the answer choices, since more than one may seem right at first.

Even if you're paying attention to the time, you may find yourself a little behind at some point. You should speed up to get back on track, but do so wisely. Don't panic; just take a few seconds less on each question until you're caught up. Don't guess without thinking, but do look through the answer choices and eliminate any you know are wrong. If you can get down to two choices, it is often worthwhile to guess from those. Once you've chosen an answer, move on and don't dwell on any that you skipped or had to hurry through. If a question was taking too long, chances are it was one of the harder ones, so you weren't as likely to get it right anyway.

On the other hand, if you find yourself getting ahead of schedule, it may be beneficial to slow down a little. The more quickly you work, the more likely you are to make a careless mistake that will affect your score. You've budgeted time for each question, so don't be afraid to spend that time. Practice an efficient but careful pace to get the most out of the time you have.

6

# Secret Key #5 – Have a Plan for Guessing

When you're taking the test, you may find yourself stuck on a question. Some of the answer choices seem better than others, but you don't see the one answer choice that is obviously correct. What do you do?

The scenario described above is very common, yet most test takers have not effectively prepared for it. Developing and practicing a plan for guessing may be one of the single most effective uses of your time as you get ready for the exam.

In developing your plan for guessing, there are three questions to address:

- When should you start the guessing process?
- How should you narrow down the choices?
- Which answer should you choose?

## When to Start the Guessing Process

Unless your plan for guessing is to select C every time (which, despite its merits, is not what we recommend), you need to leave yourself enough time to apply your answer elimination strategies. Since you have a limited amount of time for each question, that means that if you're going to give yourself the best shot at guessing correctly, you have to decide quickly whether or not you will guess.

Of course, the best-case scenario is that you don't have to guess at all, so first, see if you can answer the question based on your knowledge of the subject and basic reasoning skills. Focus on the key words in the question and try to jog your memory of related topics. Give yourself a chance to bring the knowledge to mind, but once you realize that you don't have (or you can't access) the knowledge you need to answer the question, it's time to start the guessing process.

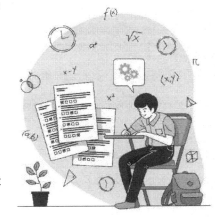

It's almost always better to start the guessing process too early than too late. It only takes a few seconds to remember something and answer the question from knowledge. Carefully eliminating wrong answer choices takes longer. Plus, going through the process of eliminating answer choices can actually help jog your memory.

**Summary**: Start the guessing process as soon as you decide that you can't answer the question based on your knowledge.

7

# How to Narrow Down the Choices

The next chapter in this book (**Test-Taking Strategies**) includes a wide range of strategies for how to approach questions and how to look for answer choices to eliminate. You will definitely want to read those carefully, practice them, and figure out which ones work best for you. Here though, we're going to address a mindset rather than a particular strategy.

Your odds of guessing an answer correctly depend on how many options you are choosing from.

| Number of options left | 5 | 4 | 3 | 2 | 1 |
|---|---|---|---|---|---|
| Odds of guessing correctly | 20% | 25% | 33% | 50% | 100% |

You can see from this chart just how valuable it is to be able to eliminate incorrect answers and make an educated guess, but there are two things that many test takers do that cause them to miss out on the benefits of guessing:

- Accidentally eliminating the correct answer
- Selecting an answer based on an impression

We'll look at the first one here, and the second one in the next section.

To avoid accidentally eliminating the correct answer, we recommend a thought exercise called **the $5 challenge**. In this challenge, you only eliminate an answer choice from contention if you are willing to bet $5 on it being wrong. Why $5? Five dollars is a small but not insignificant amount of money. It's an amount you could afford to lose but wouldn't want to throw away. And while losing

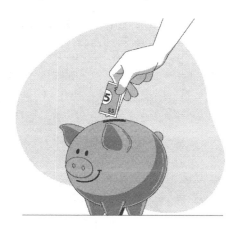

$5 once might not hurt too much, doing it twenty times will set you back $100. In the same way, each small decision you make—eliminating a choice here, guessing on a question there—won't by itself impact your score very much, but when you put them all together, they can make a big difference. By holding each answer choice elimination decision to a higher standard, you can reduce the risk of accidentally eliminating the correct answer.

The $5 challenge can also be applied in a positive sense: If you are willing to bet $5 that an answer choice *is* correct, go ahead and mark it as correct.

**Summary**: Only eliminate an answer choice if you are willing to bet $5 that it is wrong.

8

# Which Answer to Choose

You're taking the test. You've run into a hard question and decided you'll have to guess. You've eliminated all the answer choices you're willing to bet $5 on. Now you have to pick an answer. Why do we even need to talk about this? Why can't you just pick whichever one you feel like when the time comes?

The answer to these questions is that if you don't come into the test with a plan, you'll rely on your impression to select an answer choice, and if you do that, you risk falling into a trap. The test writers know that everyone who takes their test will be guessing on some of the questions, so they intentionally write wrong answer choices to seem plausible. You still have to pick an answer though, and if the wrong answer choices are designed to look right, how can you ever be sure that you're not falling for their trap? The best solution we've found to this dilemma is to take the decision out of your hands entirely. Here is the process we recommend:

**Once you've eliminated any choices that you are confident (willing to bet $5) are wrong, select the first remaining choice as your answer.**

Whether you choose to select the first remaining choice, the second, or the last, the important thing is that you use some preselected standard. Using this approach guarantees that you will not be enticed into selecting an answer choice that looks right, because you are not basing your decision on how the answer choices look.

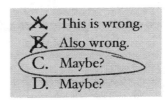

This is not meant to make you question your knowledge. Instead, it is to help you recognize the difference between your knowledge and your impressions. There's a huge difference between thinking an answer is right because of what you know, and thinking an answer is right because it looks or sounds like it should be right.

**Summary**: To ensure that your selection is appropriately random, make a predetermined selection from among all answer choices you have not eliminated.

# Test-Taking Strategies

This section contains a list of test-taking strategies that you may find helpful as you work through the test. By taking what you know and applying logical thought, you can maximize your chances of answering any question correctly!

It is very important to realize that every question is different and every person is different: no single strategy will work on every question, and no single strategy will work for every person. That's why we've included all of them here, so you can try them out and determine which ones work best for different types of questions and which ones work best for you.

## Question Strategies

### ☑ READ CAREFULLY

Read the question and the answer choices carefully. Don't miss the question because you misread the terms. You have plenty of time to read each question thoroughly and make sure you understand what is being asked. Yet a happy medium must be attained, so don't waste too much time. You must read carefully and efficiently.

### ☑ CONTEXTUAL CLUES

Look for contextual clues. If the question includes a word you are not familiar with, look at the immediate context for some indication of what the word might mean. Contextual clues can often give you all the information you need to decipher the meaning of an unfamiliar word. Even if you can't determine the meaning, you may be able to narrow down the possibilities enough to make a solid guess at the answer to the question.

### ☑ PREFIXES

If you're having trouble with a word in the question or answer choices, try dissecting it. Take advantage of every clue that the word might include. Prefixes and suffixes can be a huge help. Usually, they allow you to determine a basic meaning. *Pre-* means before, *post-* means after, *pro-* is positive, *de-* is negative. From prefixes and suffixes, you can get an idea of the general meaning of the word and try to put it into context.

### ☑ HEDGE WORDS

Watch out for critical hedge words, such as *likely, may, can, sometimes, often, almost, mostly, usually, generally, rarely,* and *sometimes*. Question writers insert these hedge phrases to cover every possibility. Often an answer choice will be wrong simply because it leaves no room for exception. Be on guard for answer choices that have definitive words such as *exactly* and *always*.

### ☑ SWITCHBACK WORDS

Stay alert for *switchbacks*. These are the words and phrases frequently used to alert you to shifts in thought. The most common switchback words are *but, although,* and *however*. Others include *nevertheless, on the other hand, even though, while, in spite of, despite,* and *regardless of*. Switchback words are important to catch because they can change the direction of the question or an answer choice.

## ⊘ FACE VALUE

When in doubt, use common sense. Accept the situation in the problem at face value. Don't read too much into it. These problems will not require you to make wild assumptions. If you have to go beyond creativity and warp time or space in order to have an answer choice fit the question, then you should move on and consider the other answer choices. These are normal problems rooted in reality. The applicable relationship or explanation may not be readily apparent, but it is there for you to figure out. Use your common sense to interpret anything that isn't clear.

# Answer Choice Strategies

## ⊘ ANSWER SELECTION

The most thorough way to pick an answer choice is to identify and eliminate wrong answers until only one is left, then confirm it is the correct answer. Sometimes an answer choice may immediately seem right, but be careful. The test writers will usually put more than one reasonable answer choice on each question, so take a second to read all of them and make sure that the other choices are not equally obvious. As long as you have time left, it is better to read every answer choice than to pick the first one that looks right without checking the others.

## ⊘ ANSWER CHOICE FAMILIES

An answer choice family consists of two (in rare cases, three) answer choices that are very similar in construction and cannot all be true at the same time. If you see two answer choices that are direct opposites or parallels, one of them is usually the correct answer. For instance, if one answer choice says that quantity $x$ increases and another either says that quantity $x$ decreases (opposite) or says that quantity $y$ increases (parallel), then those answer choices would fall into the same family. An answer choice that doesn't match the construction of the answer choice family is more likely to be incorrect. Most questions will not have answer choice families, but when they do appear, you should be prepared to recognize them.

## ⊘ ELIMINATE ANSWERS

Eliminate answer choices as soon as you realize they are wrong, but make sure you consider all possibilities. If you are eliminating answer choices and realize that the last one you are left with is also wrong, don't panic. Start over and consider each choice again. There may be something you missed the first time that you will realize on the second pass.

## ⊘ AVOID FACT TRAPS

Don't be distracted by an answer choice that is factually true but doesn't answer the question. You are looking for the choice that answers the question. Stay focused on what the question is asking for so you don't accidentally pick an answer that is true but incorrect. Always go back to the question and make sure the answer choice you've selected actually answers the question and is not merely a true statement.

## ⊘ EXTREME STATEMENTS

In general, you should avoid answers that put forth extreme actions as standard practice or proclaim controversial ideas as established fact. An answer choice that states the "process should be used in certain situations, if…" is much more likely to be correct than one that states the "process should be discontinued completely." The first is a calm rational statement and doesn't even make a definitive, uncompromising stance, using a hedge word *if* to provide wiggle room, whereas the second choice is far more extreme.

### ⊘ Benchmark

As you read through the answer choices and you come across one that seems to answer the question well, mentally select that answer choice. This is not your final answer, but it's the one that will help you evaluate the other answer choices. The one that you selected is your benchmark or standard for judging each of the other answer choices. Every other answer choice must be compared to your benchmark. That choice is correct until proven otherwise by another answer choice beating it. If you find a better answer, then that one becomes your new benchmark. Once you've decided that no other choice answers the question as well as your benchmark, you have your final answer.

### ⊘ Predict the Answer

Before you even start looking at the answer choices, it is often best to try to predict the answer. When you come up with the answer on your own, it is easier to avoid distractions and traps because you will know exactly what to look for. The right answer choice is unlikely to be word-for-word what you came up with, but it should be a close match. Even if you are confident that you have the right answer, you should still take the time to read each option before moving on.

## General Strategies

### ⊘ Tough Questions

If you are stumped on a problem or it appears too hard or too difficult, don't waste time. Move on! Remember though, if you can quickly check for obviously incorrect answer choices, your chances of guessing correctly are greatly improved. Before you completely give up, at least try to knock out a couple of possible answers. Eliminate what you can and then guess at the remaining answer choices before moving on.

### ⊘ Check Your Work

Since you will probably not know every term listed and the answer to every question, it is important that you get credit for the ones that you do know. Don't miss any questions through careless mistakes. If at all possible, try to take a second to look back over your answer selection and make sure you've selected the correct answer choice and haven't made a costly careless mistake (such as marking an answer choice that you didn't mean to mark). This quick double check should more than pay for itself in caught mistakes for the time it costs.

### ⊘ Pace Yourself

It's easy to be overwhelmed when you're looking at a page full of questions; your mind is confused and full of random thoughts, and the clock is ticking down faster than you would like. Calm down and maintain the pace that you have set for yourself. Especially as you get down to the last few minutes of the test, don't let the small numbers on the clock make you panic. As long as you are on track by monitoring your pace, you are guaranteed to have time for each question.

### ⊘ Don't Rush

It is very easy to make errors when you are in a hurry. Maintaining a fast pace in answering questions is pointless if it makes you miss questions that you would have gotten right otherwise. Test writers like to include distracting information and wrong answers that seem right. Taking a little extra time to avoid careless mistakes can make all the difference in your test score. Find a pace that allows you to be confident in the answers that you select.

## ⊘ KEEP MOVING

Panicking will not help you pass the test, so do your best to stay calm and keep moving. Taking deep breaths and going through the answer elimination steps you practiced can help to break through a stress barrier and keep your pace.

# Final Notes

The combination of a solid foundation of content knowledge and the confidence that comes from practicing your plan for applying that knowledge is the key to maximizing your performance on test day. As your foundation of content knowledge is built up and strengthened, you'll find that the strategies included in this chapter become more and more effective in helping you quickly sift through the distractions and traps of the test to isolate the correct answer.

Now that you're preparing to move forward into the test content chapters of this book, be sure to keep your goal in mind. As you read, think about how you will be able to apply this information on the test. If you've already seen sample questions for the test and you have an idea of the question format and style, try to come up with questions of your own that you can answer based on what you're reading. This will give you valuable practice applying your knowledge in the same ways you can expect to on test day.

**Good luck and good studying!**

# Safety and Compliance

## OSHA AND SDS

OSHA stands for Occupational Safety and Health Administration. It is an organization designed to assure the safety and health of workers by setting and enforcing standards; providing training, outreach, and education; establishing partnerships; and encouraging continual improvement in workplace safety and health.

SDS (formerly MSDS) stands for Safety Data Sheets. These sheets are the result of the "Right to Know" Law also known as the OSHA's HazCom Standard. This law requires chemical manufacturers to supply SDS sheets on any products that have a hazardous warning label. These sheets contain information on precautionary as well as emergency information about the product.

## VARIOUS AGENCIES AND THEIR RESPONSIBILITIES

National Accrediting Agency for Clinical Laboratory Sciences - The agency responsible for approving and accrediting clinical laboratory science and similar healthcare professional education programs.

College of American Pathologists - The primary organization for board-certified pathologists serving to represent the interests of the public, as well as pathologists and their patients by fostering excellence in the pathology and laboratory medicine practice.

The Joint Commission - A large organization that aims to improve the quality of care provided to patients through implementing healthcare accreditation standards and other supportive services aimed at improving the performance of healthcare organizations

## HIPAA AND CONFIDENTIALITY

The **Health Insurance Portability and Accountability Act** (HIPAA) addresses the rights of the individual related to confidentiality of health information. Healthcare providers must not release any information or documentation about a patient's condition or treatment without consent, as the individual has the right to determine who has access to personal information. Personal information about the patient is considered protected health information (PHI) and consists of any identifying or personal information about the patient, such as health history, condition, or treatments in any form, and any documentation, including electronic, verbal, or written. Personal information can be shared with spouse, legal guardians, those with durable power of attorney for the patient, and those involved in care of the patient, such as physicians, without a specific release, but the patient should always be consulted if personal information is to be discussed with others present to ensure there is no objection. Failure to comply with HIPAA regulations can make one liable for legal action.

## REGULATORY BODIES GOVERNING CODING AND BILLING

**CPT codes,** developed by the American Medical Association (AMA), define those licensed to provide services and describe medical and surgical treatments, diagnostics, and procedures done on an outpatient basis. The use of CPT codes is mandated by both CMS and HIPAA to provide a uniform language and to aid research. These codes are used primarily for billing purposes for insurances

15

(public and private). HHS has designed CPT codes as part of the national standard for electronic healthcare transactions:

- Category I: Identify a procedure or service.
- Category II: Identify performance measures, including diagnostic procedures.
- Category III: Identify temporary codes for technology and data collection.

**ICD-10 codes** are the tenth version of the WHO's International Statistical Classification of Diseases and Related Health Problems (ICD) codes and include ICD-10-CM, which codes for diagnosis, and ICD-10-PCS, which codes for inpatient procedures. ICD codes were developed by the World Health Organization. Use of these codes is mandated by CMS. Because insurance companies use the same coding systems as CMS, these codes are used across healthcare.

### ROUTES BIOLOGICAL HAZARDS MAY TAKE TO ENTER THE BODY

The following are the routes that biological hazards may take to enter the body:

- Airborne (through the nasal passage into the lungs)
- Ingestion (by eating)
- Broken Skin
- Percutaneous (through intact skin)
- Mucosal (through the lining of the mouth and nose)

## HEPATITIS B

Hepatitis B virus and its exposure hazards are discussed below:

- Sexually transmitted disease, also transmitted with body fluids and some individual may be symptom free but still be carriers.
- Condoms are not proved to prevent the spread of this disease.
- Symptoms: Jaundice, Dark Urine, Malaise, Joint pain, Fever, Fatigue
- Tests: Decreased albumin levels, + antibodies and antigen, Increased levels of transaminase
- Treatment: Monitor for changes in the liver. Recombinant alpha interferon in some cases. Transplant necessary if liver failure occurs.
- Prevention: Series of 3 Hepatitis B Vaccinations: an initial dose, a dose 1 month later and a final dose 6 months after the initial dose.
- HBV is the most common laboratory-associated infection.

## HEPATITIS D

The hepatitis D virus and its exposure hazards are discussed below:

- Usually acquired with HBV as a co-infection or super infection
- Signs and Symptoms: jaundice, fatigue, abdominal pain, loss of appetite, nausea, vomiting, joint pain, dark (tea colored) urine
- Transmission: Occurs when blood from an infected person enters the body of a person who is not immune. By sharing drugs, needles, or "works" when "shooting" drugs; through needle sticks or sharps exposures on the job; or from an infected mother to her baby during birth.
- Treatment: Acute HDV infection - Supportive care. Chronic HDV infection interferon-alfa, liver transplant

- Prevention: Hepatitis B vaccination. HBV-HDV co-infection - pre- or post-exposure prophylaxis (hepatitis B immune globulin or vaccine) to prevent HBV infection. HBV-HDV superinfection - education to reduce risk behaviors among persons with chronic HBV infection.

## TRANSMISSION OF HIV

The following are ways that HIV can be transmitted from an infected person to an uninfected one:

- Unprotected sexual contact. Direct blood contact, including injection drug needles, blood transfusions, accidents in health care settings or certain blood products. Mother to baby (before or during birth, or through breast milk)
- Sexual intercourse (vaginal and anal): In the genitals and the rectum, HIV may infect the mucous membranes directly or enter through cuts and sores caused during intercourse (many of which would be unnoticed).
- Oral sex (mouth-penis, mouth-vagina): The mouth is an inhospitable environment for HIV (in semen, vaginal fluid or blood), meaning the risk of HIV transmission through the throat, gums, and oral membranes is lower than through vaginal or anal membranes. There are however, documented cases where HIV was transmitted orally. Sharing injection needles: An injection needle can pass blood directly from one person's bloodstream to another. It is a very efficient way to transmit a blood-borne virus.
- Mother to Child: It is possible for an HIV-infected mother to pass the virus directly before or during birth, or through breast milk. The following "bodily fluids" are NOT infectious: Saliva, Tears, Sweat, Feces, Urine

## CHAIN OF INFECTION

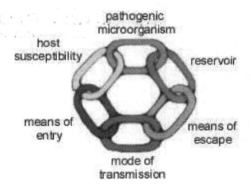

## INFECTION CONTROL METHODS

The first line of defense in infection control is hand washing. Protective Clothing is an important aspect of infection control. This includes Masks, Goggles, Face Shields, Respirators, Gowns, Lab Coats, and Gloves. The precautions that are used depend on the infection. Isolation procedures are also used this includes protective isolation or reverse isolation. In protective isolation, the patients are isolated to prevent them from getting an infection i.e. patients receiving chemotherapy. In reverse isolation, the patients are isolated to prevent others from getting their infection or disease i.e. patients with tuberculosis. Universal Precautions are used with all patients. This means do not touch or use anything that has the patient's body fluid on it without a barrier and assume that all body fluid of a patient is infectious.

## PUTTING ON AND REMOVING PROTECTIVE CLOTHING

A healthcare worker puts on the protective gown first being sure not to touch the outside of the gown. The mask in put on next. Gloves are applied last and secured over the cuffs of the gown. A healthcare worker removes the gloves first. They are removed by grasping one glove at the wrist and pulling it inside out off the hand and holding it in the gloved hand. The second glove is removed by placing your uncovered hands fingers under the edge of the glove being careful not to touch the outside of the glove and rolling it down inside out over the glove grasped in your hand. The first glove ends up inside of the second glove. Next, slide arms out of the gown and then fold the gown with the outside folded in away from the body so that the contaminated side is folded inwardly. Dispose of properly. Finally, remove the mask by touching the strings only. Always wash hands after glove removal.

## BIOHAZARD SYMBOL

## CLEANING UP SMALL BLOOD SPILLS

The best way to clean a small blood spill is to absorb the blood with a paper towel or gauze pad. Then disinfect area with a disinfectant. Soap and water is not a disinfectant nor is alcohol. Never scrape a dry spill; this may cause an aerosol of infectious organisms. If blood is dried, use the disinfectant to moisten the dried blood. *1:10 dilution of sodium hypochlorite (household bleach)*

## GENERAL KNOWLEDGE OF FIRE SAFETY

Fire requires three components to occur. They are called the fire triangle and include fuel, oxygen, and heat when a chemical source is included it forms the fire tetrahedron. In the event of a fire remember these two acronyms, RACE and PASS. RACE describes the steps for dealing with a fire. "R" stands for Rescue (rescue patients and co-workers from danger.) "A" stands for alarm (sound the alarm and alert those around you.) "C" stands for confine (confine a fire by closing the doors and windows.) "E" stands for extinguish (use the nearest fire extinguisher to put out the fire. PASS describes how to use a fire extinguisher to put out a fire. "P" stands for pull the pin. "A" stands for aim at the fire. "S" stands for squeeze the trigger. "S" stands for sweep the base of the fire. Fires are broken down into four classes. Class A fires involve ordinary combustible materials. Class B fires involve flammable liquids, Class C involves electrical fires, and Class D involves combustible metals.

## DEMING'S 14 POINTS FOR QUALITY IMPROVEMENT

1. Create and communicate to all employees a statement of the quality philosophy of the company.
2. Adopt this philosophy.
3. Build quality into a product throughout production.
4. End the practice of awarding business on the basis of price tag alone; build a long-term relationship based on established loyalty and trust.
5. Work to constantly improve quality and productivity.
6. Institute on-the-job quality training.
7. Teach and institute leadership to improve all job functions.

8. Drive out fear; create trust.
9. Strive to reduce inter- and intradepartmental conflicts.
10. Eliminate slogans and targets; instead, focus on the system and morale.
11. Eliminate numerical quotas for production and management. Substitute leadership methods for improvement.
12. Remove barriers that rob people of pride in their work.
13. Educate with self-improvement programs.
14. Include everyone in the company to accomplish the transformation.

## PATIENT CONSENTS

The types of patient consents needed to do a procedure are discussed below:

- Informed Consent - a competent person gives voluntary permission for a medical procedure after receiving adequate information about the risk of, methods used and consequences of the procedure
- Expressed Consent - permission given by patient verbally or in writing for a procedure
- Implied Consent - the patient's actions gives permission for the procedure without verbal or written consent for example going to the emergency room or holding out arm when told need to draw blood.
- HIV Consent - special permission given to administer a test for detecting the human immunodeficiency virus.
- Parental Consent for Minors - a parent or a legal guardian must give permission for procedures administered to underage patients depending on the state law may range from 18 to 21 years old.

## SCOPE OF PRACTICE AND ETHICAL STANDARDS RELATED TO PRACTICE OF PHLEBOTOMY

The **scope of practice** encompasses those duties and procedures that the person's training, licensure and/or certification, has prepared the person to undertake. The phlebotomist and other laboratory professionals must adhere to the **code of ethics** developed by the American Society for Clinical Laboratory Sciences (ASCLS):

- Duty to patient: This is the primary focus and depends on being honest, showing respect for the patient, and providing a high standard of care
- Duty to colleagues and profession: The phlebotomist and laboratory professionals must establish an honest and cooperative working relationship with colleagues and work to improve personal practice and to advance the profession,
- Duty to society: The phlebotomist and laboratory professionals must comply with laws and regulations and serve as patient advocates.
- Pledge: The phlebotomist and laboratory professionals pledge to carry out the duties outlines in the code of ethics, beginning with placing the welfare of the patient before that of self.

## AMERICANS WITH DISABILITIES ACT

The 1990 **Americans with Disabilities Act (ADA)** is civil rights legislation that provides the disabled, including those with mental impairment, access to employment and the community. The ADA covers not only obvious disabilities but also disorders such as arthritis, seizure disorders, cardiovascular and respiratory disorders. Communities must provide transportation services for the disabled, including accommodation for wheelchairs. Public facilities (schools, museums, physician's offices, post offices, restaurants, hospitals, laboratories) must be accessible with ramps and elevators as needed. Telecommunications must also be accessible through devices or accommodations for the deaf and blind. Laboratories must accommodate those with disabilities and may need to provide sign language translators or other methods of communicating with patients when necessary. Some patients, such as those who are legally blind, may have service animals (only a dog), and these animals must be allowed to accompany the person in all public areas. Comfort animals are not covered by the ADA.

## CONVERSION CHART OF METRIC TO ENGLISH

|  | Metrix | English |
|---|---|---|
| **Distance** | meter | 3.3 feet |
| **Weight** | gram | 0.0022 pounds |
| **Volume** | liter | 1.06 quarts |

## ROMAN NUMERALS

The following Roman numerals equal the Arabic numbers.

$$I = 1$$
$$V = 5$$
$$X = 10$$
$$L = 50$$
$$C = 100$$
$$D = 500$$
$$M = 1000$$

## MILITARY AND CIVILIAN TIME

| Military | = | Civilian |  | Military | = | Civilian |
|---|---|---|---|---|---|---|
| 0001 | = | 12:01 AM |  | 1200 | = | 12 Noon |
| 0100 | = | 1:00 AM |  | 1300 | = | 1:00 PM |
| 0200 | = | 2:00 AM |  | 1400 | = | 2:00 PM |
| 0300 | = | 3:00 AM |  | 1500 | = | 3:00 PM |
| 0400 | = | 4:00 AM |  | 1600 | = | 4:00 PM |
| 0500 | = | 5:00 AM |  | 1700 | = | 5:00 PM |
| 0600 | = | 6:00 AM |  | 1800 | = | 6:00 PM |
| 0700 | = | 7:00 AM |  | 1900 | = | 7:00 PM |
| 0800 | = | 8:00 AM |  | 2000 | = | 8:00 PM |
| 0900 | = | 9:00 AM |  | 2100 | = | 9:00 PM |
| 1000 | = | 10:00 AM |  | 2200 | = | 10:00 PM |
| 1100 | = | 11:00 AM |  | 2300 | = | 11:00 PM |
| 1200 | = | 12 Noon |  | 0000 | = | 12 Midnight |

## EQUATIONS TO CHANGE FAHRENHEIT TO CELSIUS AND CELSIUS TO FAHRENHEIT

Fahrenheit into Celsius

$$C = (F - 32) \times 5/9$$

Celsius into Fahrenheit

$$F = (C \times 9/5) + 32$$

## Formula to Convert Pounds into Kilograms

$$Kilograms = (Pounds \times 0.4536)$$

## Equation to Determine Percentage

$$(amount \div total) \times 100 = percentage$$

## Dilution of 1:100 in a Blood Culture Dilution

The dilution of 1:100 means that there is 1mL of blood and 99mL of media for every 100 mL of blood culture specimen.

## Approximating Liters of Blood in Normal Adults

The average adult has 70 mL of blood per kilogram of weight. In the United States, a person weigh is usually recorded in pounds. You will need to convert the pounds into kilograms by using the conversion factor of 0.454. The person's weight in kilograms is multiplied by 70 which is the average mL of blood per kilogram. Then divide that number by 1000 to convert the mL into Liters.

## Approximating Liters of Blood in Infants

The average infant has 100 mL of blood per kilogram of weight. If an infant's weight is given in pounds it must be converted to kilograms using the conversion factor of 0.454. That number is then multiplied by 100 which is the average mL of blood per kilogram in an infant. Then divide that number by 1000 to convert the mL into liters.

## Terms

**CLSI**: The <u>Clinical and Laboratory Standards Institute</u> provides standards for a wide range of performance and testing and covers all types of laboratory functions and microbiology. These standards are used as a basis for quality control procedures. Standards include: Labeling, security/information technology, toxicology/drug testing, statistical quality control, and performance standards for various types of antimicrobial susceptibility testing.

**CLIA**: In the United States, all laboratory testing, except for research, is regulated by the CMS (Centers for Medicare and Medicaid) through <u>Clinical Laboratory Improvement Amendments.</u> CLIA is implemented through the Division of Laboratory Services and serves approximately 244,000 laboratories. Laboratories receiving reimbursement from CMS must meet CLIA standards, which ensure that laboratory testing will be accurate and procedures followed properly.

**CDC**: <u>The Centers for Disease Control and Prevention</u> is a federal agency that supports health promotion, prevention, and health preparedness. The CDC partners with CMS and the FDA in supporting CLIA programs.

**Communicable Infection**: An illness caused by the direct or indirect transmission of a specific infectious agent or the toxins it produces from an infected person, animal, or inanimate host to a susceptible body; indirect transmission can be via a vector, intermediate plant or animal host, or the inanimate environment.

**Nosocomial Infection**: Hospital-acquired illness not resulting from the original reason for the patient to be admitted.

**Tort**: An injury or wrong committed, either with or without force, to the person or property of another, for which civil liability may be imposed.

**Assault**: The touching of another person with an intent to harm, without that person's consent, A willful attempt to illegally inflict injury on or threaten a person

**Malpractice**: A lawsuit raised against a professional for injury or loss resulting from negligence on the part of the professional in rendering services.

**Negligence**: Failure to perform or act with the prudence expected by a reasonable person in the same circumstance.

**Vicarious liability**: When a person is held responsible for the tort of another even though the person being held responsible may not have done anything wrong. This is often the case with employers who are held vicariously liable for the damages caused by their employees.

**Breach of confidentiality**: Occurs when information that should be kept secret, with access limited to appropriate persons, is given to an inappropriate person

**Fraud**: An intentional perversion of truth; deceitful practice or device resorted to with intent to deprive another of property or other right.

**Gram**: Basic metric unit of weight

**Meter**: Basic metric unit of distance

**Liter**: Basic metric unit of volume

**Risk Management**: System that involves identifying and reducing situations that pose unnecessary risk to employees or patients by following specific procedures and by adequately educating employees on policies and procedures adopted by the facility.

**Quality Control**: A series of checks and control measures that ensure that a uniform excellence of service is provided

**Quality Assurance**: The system utilizing quality reviews of services and the taking of any corrective actions to remove or improve any deficiencies

## SAMPLE QUESTIONS

Discuss how the following situations violate patients' rights.

1. A patient is told that he will be restrained if he doesn't stop moving so that a specimen can be collected.
2. A co-worker tells you in the hospital cafeteria that your patient, Mr. Louis, has HIV.
3. An unsupervised 10-year-old refuses to have his blood drawn; a co-worker helps hold him down while you draw the blood.
4. You forget to put a needle in the sharp's container and a 2-year-old gets stuck.

## ANSWERS

1. The patient has been threatened with the fear of restraint. This falls into the category of assault.
2. This is a breach of confidentiality. The information has been given to you in an inappropriate location. Someone who knows Mr. Louis may have overheard the information exchange. All information about a patient should be considered confidential.

3. If the parents are not there to consent to a blood draw, this may be considered assault and battery.
4. This is a case of negligence. You were responsible for putting the needle into the sharp's container and harm was done to the child as a result of your action.

What are the Fahrenheit and Celsius degrees for the following?

1. Normal body temperature
2. Room temperature
3. Boiling point of water
4. Freezing point of water

ANSWERS

| Normal body temperature | 98.6 °F | 37 °C |
|---|---|---|
| Room temperature | 68-77 °F | 20-25 °C |
| Boiling point of water | 212 °F | 100 °C |
| Freezing point of water | 32 °F | 0 °C |

Determine if each of the following is true or false:

1. CC and mL are used interchangeably in the laboratory.
2. Five teaspoons are equal to one milliliter.
3. A millimeter is 1/1000 of a meter
4. XII is the Roman numeral form of the Arabic number 12.

ANSWERS

All of the statements are true.

# Patient Preparation

## REQUISITION

The **requisition** is the form in which the tests a patient is having are entered, and the requisition then becomes part of the patient's permanent record. Requisition forms may be filled out manually or electronically. Electronic requisitions often automatically print out the labels with barcodes that will be affixed to the collection tubes. Required elements for a requisition form include:

- Name of ordering healthcare provider.
- Patient's full name.
- Patient's ID number (patient number if an inpatient).
- Room number if inpatient.
- Patient's birthdate.
- Test to be performed.
- Test priorities.
- Date and specific directions for test (such as "stat," or "fasting").
- Billing information and codes as needed.
- Allergies or any special precautions ("latex allergy," "sensitive to adhesive").

The laboratory professional should carefully check the requisition to make sure it is complete, verify the patient's identification before proceeding with sample collections, ensure any test requirements, such as "fasting," have been met, verify the date, and determine the priorities for collection.

## PATIENT CONSENT AND RIGHT TO REFUSE TREATMENT

Patients should give **informed consent** prior to any procedures, including laboratory tests. That is, the patient should understand the purpose, the risks, and the benefits as well as the method. Hospitalized patients sign a general consent form that covers most routine laboratory tests although some tests, such as HIV tests, may require a separate consent form. While consent may be verbal or in writing, written consent provides the most protection for the healthcare provider. **Expressed content** is consent that is given verbally or in writing. In some cases, such as in emergency care, **implied consent** is assumed, but laws vary from one state to another. Whenever a laboratory sample is obtained from a patient, the patient should first be advised the type of test and the purpose. Competent adult patients have the **right to refuse any treatment**, even if it is lifesaving. If a patient refuses a test (for example, a blood draw), the phlebotomist must immediately stop, inform the ordering healthcare provider, and document the refusal.

## IDENTIFYING PATIENT PRIOR TO SAMPLE COLLECTION

The first step in any blood draw or laboratory procedure for inpatients and outpatients should be to properly **identify the patient**, utilizing at least two forms of identification. Alert and responsive patients (or parents of a minor) may be asked to give their names and birthdates:

1. Introduce yourself to the patient and explain your purpose.
2. Check ID band against information provided by patient/caregiver/parent.
3. Match specimen labeling to information on ID band and label immediately with barcode labeler or permanent ink.
4. Check ankles for ID band if missing from wrists.

5. Consider only ID bands actually on the patient as valid (not on bedside stand/bed) except in special circumstances (severe burns of extremities). Verify ID with nurse in these cases.
6. If armband missing, procure armband and secure on patient before procedure.
7. Ask outpatients for picture ID and verify name and birthdate verbally if possible.
8. For emergent situations (unconscious patient in ED), check "Jane/John Doe" ID as per protocol.
9. For call reports, verify patient's name, birthdate, and ID number.

## COMMUNICATING WITH PATIENT DURING SAMPLE COLLECTION

The first thing a phlebotomist should do before **collecting a sample** is to make introductions to the patient, check the patient's identification (often through asking name and birthdate and checking wristband), and explain the purpose of the visit: "My name is John Doe, and I'm going to draw blood for the thyroid tests that your physician has ordered." The phlebotomist should make a point of explaining actions, "I'm going to take a look at the veins in your arms" and should ask if the patient has a preference, "Where do you prefer to have blood drawn?" if possible. If patients are quite nervous or frightened, especially young children, chatting with them briefly may help to distract them. The phlebotomist should remain professional and confident throughout the procedure and avoid making statements that may not be true, "You will barely feel this," because this violates the trust between the patient and phlebotomist.

## PATIENT INTERVIEWING STRATEGIES AND TECHNIQUES

**Interviewing strategies and techniques** include:

- Establishing rapport with the patient: Take time to make introductions and chat for a moment, especially if the patient appears anxious.
- Positioning within the patient's field of vision: Position in face-to-face position so that the patient does not have to look up or down during the interview.
- Avoiding medical jargon: Ask questions and respond in language that the patient is familiar with and explain any unclear terms used.
- Ensuring patient privacy/confidentiality: Be alert to the surroundings and make sure that questions and patient's responses remain confidential and cannot be overheard.
- Observing body language: Note nonverbal communication (eye contact, gestures, position, expressions, proxemics) for clues about the patient's emotional state and feelings.
- Asking open-ended questions: Avoid questions that can be answered with simple "yes" or "no" as much as possible.
- Allowing patient time to respond: Do not look at a watch, fidget, or appear in a hurry.
- Practicing active listening: Make eye contact, nod, respond, and pay attention when patient speaks.
- Respecting cultural differences: Avoid judgmental attitudes or comments.

## PRIORITIZATION OF SPECIMEN COLLECTION AND RESULTS

The nomenclature and scheme for the prioritization of specimen collection and results are as follows:

| Priority | Discussion |
|---|---|
| 1. STAT, Med. Emergency, Immediate | Patient critical or results needed immediately. Tests include glucose, cardiac enzymes, hemoglobin and hematocrit, and electrolytes. Collect sample immediately and alert laboratory technicians. STAT orders from ED usually have priority over inpatient STAT orders. |
| 2. Timed specimen | Must be obtained as close to specified time as possible to ensure meaningful results. Tests include 2-hour PP GTT, cortisol, blood cultures, cardiac enzymes. Note exact time of collection on sample. |
| 3. ASAP (as soon as possible), Preop, and Postop | Patient is in serious but not critical condition. Tests include hemoglobin and hematocrit, electrolytes, and glucose. Preop collected before surgery to verify suitability (CBC, platelet function, hemoglobin, hematocrit, PTT, type and crossmatch) and postop to assess condition (hemoglobin, hematocrit). Some patients (preop) may be NPO. |
| 4. Fasting | Verify fasting before collection. Tests include glucose, cholesterol, triglycerides. |
| 5. Routine | Collect when possible but no urgency because used to monitor condition or establish diagnosis. Tests include CBC and chemistry panels. |

## TESTING REQUIREMENTS FOR FASTING, MEDICATIONS, AND BASAL STATE

Some tests need to be carried out during a patient's **basal state**, which is the state the body is in when the patient awakens in the morning after 12 hours of fasting (no nutritional intake although water is usually allowed). In practice, patients are usually asked to fast for 8 to 12 hours, depending on the test. In addition to fasting, patients should be advised to avoiding smoking, chewing any kind of gum, or exercising as these may alter the patient's basal state and affect test results. In some cases, patients may be asked to withhold alcohol or drugs for a period of time (often the day before the test). Tests that are usually done after fasting include:

- Glucose: 8 hours.
- Triglycerides: 9 to 12 hours.
- Lipids: 9 to 12 hours.
- Renal function tests: 8 to 12 hours.
- Vitamin B-12 test: 6 to 8 hours.
- Basic/Comprehensive metabolic panels: 10 to 12 hours.
- GGT: 8 hours.
- Iron levels: 12 hours.

## BLOOD VOLUME REQUIREMENTS

Syringes and collection tubes vary in size. Vacutainer tubes are available in multiple sizes, including pediatric, and are selected according to the usual volume needed for the specified tests. Tubes have **maximum and minimum fill** lines, and each tube specifies a draw volume, so the phlebotomist must verify this draw volume before collecting a sample, and the sample should be within 10% +/- of this draw volume if possible. Overfilling can be a problem with additives because it changes the

26

ratio of additive to sample. Underfilling may result in a sample inadequate for testing. Typical minimum fills (but may vary according to tube size and type of tube):

- CBC and differential: 0.25 to 0.5 mL; pediatric, 1.5 mL.
- Coagulation: 2.5 m; pediatric 1.8 mL.
- Blood cultures: Varies widely, larger specimen (up to 20 mL) preferred but if <1 mL, only the aerobic tube should be filled.
- CMP: 1.2 mL.
- Electrolytes: 0.7 mL.
- Therapeutic drug levels: 0.5 mL.

## BLOOD COLLECTION PROCEDURES

**Anchoring a vein** involves stretching the skin to provide a taut surface and securing the vein to minimize moving and rolling during puncture. When the puncture site is the antecubital area, the thumb should be placed one to two inches below the antecubital area pulling the tissue distally with the other fingers wrapped about the back of the arm to secure the arm. It's important to avoid a C-hold with the thumb below and index finger above the puncture site because this poses a risk of accidental needlestick if the patient jerks the arm way. If veins on the back of the hand are used, then the patient's hand should be grasped right below the knuckles, the patient's fingers bent, and the skin on the top of the hand stretched taut with the thumb. Most **needles** are inserted bevel up at an angle of 15° to 30°, depending on the vein depth, in a proximal direction. A slight decrease in resistance (often characterized as a "pop") is felt when the needle enters the vein.

## LOCATING VEINS THAT ARE DIFFICULT TO VISUALIZE OR FEEL

When **veins are difficult to visualize or feel**, different techniques may be utilized:

- Massage: Gently massaging the arm starting at the wrist and moving proximally to the venipuncture site after applying the tourniquet may help veins stand out; however, excessive massaging may cause some change in results.
- Heat application: Applying a heating pad or warm moist compress to the site for 5 minutes may help to distend the vein by causing vasodilation, making the vein easier to locate.
- Fist pumping: After the tourniquet is applied, the patient should be asked to make a fist as this helps the veins to appear more prominent. However, repeatedly pumping the fist should be avoided because this may alter some test results (potassium, phosphate), and the movement may make the vein harder to locate.
- Positioning: Lowering the arm to a dependent position (such as over the side of the bed) may help to fill the veins and make them easier to locate. Rotating the arm may help to locate a vein.

## PROPER ANTISEPTIC AGENT FOR COMMON PHLEBOTOMY TESTS

**Antiseptics** inhibit organisms but do not kill all of them; however, the disinfectants that are better able to kill organisms are unsafe to use of skin. A number of different antiseptics can be used for skin preparation for common phlebotomy tests:

- Isopropyl alcohol 70%: This is the most commonly used antiseptic as it is tolerated by most individuals and has good antiseptic qualities. It is usually supplied in individually wrapped pads.
- Ethyl alcohol: Generally needs to be a higher concentration and left on for a longer period of time than isopropyl alcohol.

27

- <u>Povidone-iodine/Tincture of iodine:</u> Used when higher order antisepsis is needed, such as for blood cultures. However, many patients are allergic to iodine, so this limits use.
- <u>Benzalkonium chloride:</u> May be used as a substitute for alcohol, such as for blood alcohol levels.
- <u>Chlorhexidine gluconate:</u> Used when higher order antisepsis is needed, such as for blood cultures, and recommended for IV catheter sites.

# Routine Blood Collections

## INITIATING PATIENT CONTACT

The following are the steps in initiating patient contact:

1. Knock on door before entering patient's room, slowly open the door and ask if it is alright to enter.
2. Look for signs on door indicating special precautions that you need to take i.e. protective clothing needed
3. Identify your name and reason for entering room
4. In the event of a physician or member of the clergy being in the room, it is not inappropriate to explain who you are and proceed to do the draw if the draw is STAT.
5. Ask the family to step out of the room.

## DRAWING BLOOD FROM SLEEPING PATIENT

Drawing blood from a sleeping patient, my startle the patient and my change testing results. Also, you or the patient could be injured as the result of the patient being startled. The appropriate action to take would be to gently say the patient's name and shake the bed (never the patient) to wake them up.

## PROPER PATIENT IDENTIFICATION

Proper patient identification is important because it can prevent a critical error like misidentifying a patient specimen which could result in harm or death to a patient. Patient identification includes asking a patient to state their name and date of birth, and then you check the identification band and the requisition to see if they match. Verbal identification should never be relied on alone although it is important since patients can be hard of hearing, ill, or mentally incompetent and may give incorrect information. Also, check the identification band since it is possible for a patient to be wearing the wrong ID band. If there is no ID band, notify the nurse and have her confirm the patient's identity and attach an ID band before the blood is drawn. If there is any discrepancy on the ID band, information given by the patient or on the requisition, a reconciliation of the discrepancy must be made before a collection is taken. More than one patient may have the same name. Usually a name alert is placed on the chart but not in all cases.

## PATIENT PREPARATION FOR GLUCOSE TOLERANCE TEST

A patient should eat balanced meals with 150 grams of carbohydrates for 3 days. They should refrain from eating 12 hours before the test as well as not smoking or chewing gum before or during the testing period.

## RESPONSIBILITY OF INFORMING PATIENTS OF PROGNOSIS

The phlebotomist's responsibility is not to inform a patient of his prognosis; this is the responsibility of the patient's physician. The phlebotomist may not know all the facts of the case and may give false and detrimental information to the patient. Encourage the patient to ask the physician about the prognosis.

When asked about a collection being drawn, do not discuss in detail what is being tested for since there can be various reasons why a test was ordered by the patient's physician. Respond to the patient that the physician has ordered these test as a part of the patient's medical care and that if they have any questions about them please ask the physician.

## ETHICAL DECISION MAKING

Steps in the ethical decision-making process are as follows:

1. Identify or determine the health problem.
2. Determine the ethical issue.
3. Obtain additional information.
4. Identify the decision maker.
5. Assess ethical and moral principles.
6. Research and consider alternative options.
7. Implement decisions as needed.
8. Assess and modify actions.

## AGE AND WEIGHT REQUIREMENTS TO DONATE BLOOD

The donor must be between the ages of 17 and 66. The donor must weigh at least 110lbs.

## EQUIPMENT FOR BLOOD COLLECTION

**Equipment needed for blood collection** includes:

- Phlebotomy cart or tray to hold equipment for easy access.
- PPI, including gloves: Latex gloves should be avoided as many patients are allergic to latex, and powdered gloves pose a risk of sample contamination. Glove liners can be used for phlebotomists that are sensitive to gloves.
- Antiseptics: Isopropyl alcohol 70%, povidone iodine, and chlorhexidine gluconate are most commonly used.
- Gauze pads and bandages: Cotton balls should not be used to apply pressure on the puncture site because they may adhere to the tissue and cause bleeding when removed.
- Vein-locating devices: If necessary and available.
- Tourniquet: Non-latex are preferable. Various sizes should be available, including extra-large for obese patients and pediatric sizes. They should be flat and about 1 inch in width. May be disposable or reusable.
- Needles, syringes, tube holders, evacuated collection tubes of various types, depending on the tests to be performed.
- Sharps container: Must be available to dispose of needles.

## NEEDLE GAUGE AND SELECTION

The gauge of a needle is a number that is inversely correlates to the diameter of the internal space of the needle for example the larger the needle the smaller the internal space of the needle and the smaller the number the larger the internal space of the needle. Since color-coding varies between manufactures, be careful of using this method to determine the gauge of a needle. When selecting a needle for venipuncture, there are several factors to consider which include the type of procedure, the condition and size of the patient's vein, and the equipment being used. The length of the needle used is determined by the depth of the vein. Keep in mind that the smaller the gauge the larger the bore. The 21-gauge needle is the standard needle used for routine venipuncture.

## NEEDLE SAFETY DEVICES

Needle safety devices protect the needle user's hand by having it remain behind the needle during use and by providing a barrier between the user's hand and the needle after use. Also, the needle safety devices are operable with using a one-handed technique and provide a permanent barrier around the contaminated needle.

## BUTTERFLY NEEDLE

If a patient, such as a child or adult who is very thin with prominent veins, requires a low needle angle for venipuncture, the best choice is probably a **winged infusion ("Butterfly") set** with syringe because the syringe is not attached to the needle, so it does not get in the way, allowing a very low angle (10° to 15°) for venipuncture as the needle can be held almost parallel to the skin. Winged needles are also useful to access hand veins and scalp veins of infants. The needle (usually 23-gauge although 25-gauge may be used if vessels are extremely small) ranges from ½ to ¾ inch in length with 12 to 15 inches of tubing to which the syringe is attached. For insertion, the "wing," which are flexible, are grasped to guide the needle. For toddlers, a 23-gauge butterfly needle is often used to draw blood from the antecubital area.

## SYRINGE SYSTEM

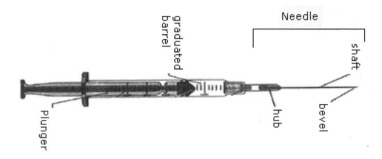

## TOURNIQUET

A tourniquet is used to aid in the collection of a blood specimen. The tourniquet is tied in such a way that it is easily removed above the venipuncture site. The purpose of the tourniquet is to slow down venous flow away from the puncture site and to not inhibit arterial flow to the puncture site. By doing this, the vein enlarges to make it easier to locate and puncture. A tourniquet should not be left on longer than 1 minute because this may change the composition of the blood and make testing inaccurate.

## BLOOD COLLECTION ADDITIVES

### ANTICOAGULANT

- EDTA
- Citrates
- Heparin
- Oxalates

### ANTIGLYCOLYTIC AGENT

- Sodium fluoride
- Lithium iodoacetate

### ADDITIVES FOUND WITH COLORED TUBE STOPPERS

- Yellow – SPS and ACD
- Red (glass tube) – no additive
- Light blue – sodium citrate
- Lavender – EDTA
- Dark Green – heparin
- Gray – potassium oxalate and sodium fluoride
- Gold –silica, thixotropic gel

- Mottled red and gray - silica, thixotropic gel

## HEPARIN

The anticoagulant heparin works by inhibiting thrombin which is required during the coagulation process. Thrombin is needed to form fibrin from fibrinogen. Thus, when thrombin is inhibited a fibrin clot is less likely to develop.

> **Review Video: Heparin – An Injectable Anti-Coagulant**
> Visit mometrix.com/academy and enter code: 127426

## COLLECTION TUBE TESTS, ADDITIVES, SPECIMEN TYPE, NUMBER OF INVERSIONS, AND DEPARTMENT

### BLACK, DARK BLUE, AND LIGHT BLUE

| Collection tube | Black | Blue (dark) | Blue (light) |
|---|---|---|---|
| Tests | ESR | Toxicology, trace metals, nutritional analysis | Coagulation |
| Additives | Sodium citrate | EDTA, heparin, or none | Sodium citrate |
| Specimen | Whole blood | Plasma or serum | Plasma |
| Inversions | 0 | Heparin or EDTA—8-10. No additive-0. | 3-4 |
| Department | Hematology | Hematology | Hematology |
| Notes | Do not invert. Fill tube completely. | Verify additive before proceeding. | Fill tube completely. |

### GOLD/TIGER-TOP/RED-GRAY, GRAY OR LIGHT GRAY, AND DARK GREEN

| Collection tube | Gold, tiger-top, red-gray | Gray, Light gray | Green (dark) |
|---|---|---|---|
| Tests | Blood chemistries, serology, immunology | Lactic acid, GTT, FBS, blood alcohol | Blood chemistry, ammonia, electrolytes, ABG |
| Additives | Clot activator and/or thixotropic gel | Iodoacetate, sodium fluoride, and/or potassium oxalate or heparin or EDTA | Heparin (sodium) |
| Specimen | Serum | Plasma | Plasma or whole blood |
| Inversions | 5-6 | 8-10 | 8-10 |
| Department | Chemistry | Chemistry | Chemistry |
| Notes | AKA serum separator tube | May need to be placed on ice. | STAT test |

### LIGHT GREEN OR GRAY/GREEN, LAVENDER, AND ORANGE OR YELLOW-GRAY

| Collection tube | Light Green, Gray/Green | Lavender | Orange, Yellow-gray |
|---|---|---|---|
| Tests | Potassium, chemistry tests | CBC, molecular tests | Chemistry tests |

32

| Collection tube | Light Green, Gray/Green | Lavender | Orange, Yellow-gray |
|---|---|---|---|
| Additives | Heparin (lithium), thixotropic gel | EDTA | Thrombin |
| Specimen | Plasma | Whole blood | Serum |
| Inversions | 8-10 | 8-10 | 8-10 |
| Department | Chemistry | Hematology | Chemistry |
| Notes | | Most common test | STAT test |

## PINK, RED (GLASS), AND RED (PLASTIC)

| Collection tube | Pink | Red (glass) | Red (plastic) |
|---|---|---|---|
| Tests | Hematology, Typing and screening | Chemistry, serology, immunology, crossmatch (for blood bank) | Chemistry, serology |
| Additives | EDTA | None | Clot activators |
| Specimen | Whole blood | Serum | Serum |
| Inversions | 8-10 | 0 | 0 |
| Department | Blood bank | Chemistry | Chemistry |
| Notes | Do not confuse pink and lavender tubes. | Specimen must rest 30 minutes. Do not confuse with plastic red tube. | Specimen must rest 30 minutes. Do not confuse with glass red tube. |

## TAN, STERILE YELLOW, AND NON-STERILE YELLOW

| Collection tube | Tan | Yellow (sterile) | Yellow (non-sterile) |
|---|---|---|---|
| Tests | Lead analysis | Blood culture | HLA, paternity test, tissue typing |
| Additives | K2 or EDTA | SPS | Acid citrate dextrose (ACD) |
| Specimen | Plasma | Whole blood | Whole blood |
| Inversions | 8-10 | 8-10 | 8-10 |
| Department | Chemistry | Microbiology | Chemistry |
| Notes | | Do not confuse with nonsterile yellow tube. | Do not confuse with sterile yellow tube. |

# PPT, SST, AND PST

All three tubes contain thixotropic gel which is a non-reactive synthetic substance that serves as an actual physical barrier between the serum and the cellular portion of a specimen after the specimen has been centrifuged. If thixotropic gel is used in tube with EDTA, it is referred to as a plasma preparation tube (PPT.) When thixotropic gel is used in serum collection tube, the gel is referred to as serum separator thus the tube and the gel are called the serum separator tube (SST.) When thixotropic gel is used in a tube with heparin, it is called plasma separator. Thus, when thixotropic gel and heparin are in a tube; the tube is called the plasma separator tube (PST.)

## BASAL STATE

The basal state is defined at the condition of the body early in the morning while the body is at rest and has been fasting for about 12 hours. For example, a patient who at dinner at 5:00PM and wakes at 5:00AM is close to his or her body's basal state.

### FACTORS INFLUENCING BASAL STATE

- Age
- Altitude
- Daily variations
- Dehydration
- Diet
- Drugs (prescription and illegal)
- Exercise
- Fever
- Gender
- Humidity
- Jaundice
- Position
- Pregnancy
- Smoking
- Stress
- Temperature

## DISINFECTANT AND ANTISEPTIC

Disinfectants are used to kill possible pathogens. They are bactericidal corrosive compounds composed of chemicals. Some disinfectants are capable of killing viruses such as HIV and HBV. These are not used on humans to disinfect skin. A common disinfectant is bleach in a 1:10 dilution. Antiseptics are chemical compounds that inhibit or prevent the growth of microorganism microbes usually applied extecrnally. Antiseptics attempt to prevent sepsis but do not necessarily kill bacteria and viruses. Antiseptics are used on human skin. Common antiseptics include70% isopropyl alcohol, betadine, and benzalkonium chloride with isopropyl alcohol being the most commonly used. Betadine is used when a sterile draw is needed.

## INVERSION

**Inversion** (the act of rotating a collection tube up and down) is carried out to mix an additive with the blood sample. Tubes without additives do not require inversions. Inversions must be done gently to thoroughly mix the additive with the sample. It's important to avoid shaking the tube or inverting too vigorously because this may result in hemolysis of the sample. If hemolysis occurs, then a number of different tests cannot be performed on the sample, including electrolyte and enzyme tests. If the inversions are done inadequately and the additive is not thoroughly mixed with the sample, microclots may develop; and these may interfere with hematology tests. If inversion of gel separation tubes does not result in thorough mixing, this may interfere with clotting. The number of inversions needed various according to the type of test and the type additive, but most additives require 8 to 10 inversions.

## POTASSIUM

Potassium is represented by the letter K. It is an electrolyte that helps maintain the body's homeostasis. The body maintains its levels of potassium in a very narrow range since too much or too little of an electrolyte can result in death if the imbalance is not corrected. The roles that potassium fills in the human body include maintain the acidic and basic balance, assisting in muscle functions, assisting with nerve conduction and maintaining osmotic pressure. Another major role that it plays involves the heart's cardiac output; it assists in this by controlling the heart rate and the heart's contraction force.

## NORMAL ARTERIAL BLOOD pH

7.35-7.45 is the normal range for arterial blood pH. Acidosis describes below normal blood pH. Alkalosis describes above normal blood pH. pH is the measure of the acidity of a solution. pH is equal to the negative logarithm of the concentration of hydrogen ions in a solution. A pH of 7 is neutral. Values less than 7 are acidic, and values greater than 7 are basic. A range of 6.5 to 7.5 is considered a neutral environment.

## INAPPROPRIATE SITE SELECTION

The following are some variables that make a site inappropriate for selection:

1. Injuries to the skin such as burns, scars, and tattoos
2. damaged veins from repeated collections or drug use
3. Swelling (edema)
4. Hematoma (Bruising
5. Mastectomy or cancer removal including skin cancer

## SELECTING EQUIPMENT AFTER FINDING COLLECTION SITE

This allows you to waste less equipment if your collection site turns out to be inappropriate for the equipment you have assembled. Also, this allows for adequate drying time for the alcohol which allows for proper cleaning of the site and reduced sting from the alcohol. A site should have a minimum drying time of 30 seconds.

## RECOMMENDED SKIN PUNCTURE SITE FOR OLDER CHILDREN AND ADULTS

The recommended site for skin puncture for this age group is the fleshy portion on the palmar surface of the distal segment of the middle or ring finger.

## FIRST DROPLET OF BLOOD OF A SKIN PUNCTURE

The first droplet of blood contains excess tissue fluid which may affect test results. Also, the alcohol residue on the skin will be wiped away with the first droplet of blood. The alcohol can hemolyze the blood specimen and keep a round droplet of blood from forming.

## PREFERRED METHOD OF RETRIEVING BLOOD FROM CHILD OR INFANT

Skin puncture is the preferred method for retrieving blood from a child or infant because children have smaller quantities of blood than adults which can lead to anemia if enough blood is drawn. Also, a child or infant may be hurt if they need to be restrained during a venipuncture. Also, infants may go into cardiac arrest if more than 10% of their blood volume is removed. If a child moves around during venipuncture, it may result in an injury to nerves, veins, and arteries.

## SAFEST PLACE FOR HEEL PUNCTURE IN INFANTS

NCCLS states that the safest areas for skin puncture in an infant are on the plantar surface of the hell, medial to the imaginary line extending from the middle of the big toe to the heel or lateral to an imaginary line extending from between the fourth and fifth toes to the heel. Deep punctures of an infant's heel can lead to osteochondritis (inflammation of the bone and cartilage) and osteomyelitis (inflammation of the bone).

## ORDER OF DRAW

Blood collection tubes must be drawn in a specific order to avoid cross-contamination of additives between tubes. The recommended order of draw is:

1. Blood culture tube (yellow-black stopper)
2. Coagulation tube (light blue stopper). If just a routine coagulation assay is the only test ordered, then a single light blue stopper tube may be drawn. If there is a concern regarding contamination by tissue fluids or thromboplastins, then one may draw a non-additive tube first, and then the light blue stopper. This sample must be filled completely to the fill line in order to be analyzed.
3. Non-additive tube (red stopper or SST)
4. Additive tubes in this order:
   o Serum separator tube (SST; red-gray, or gold, stopper). Contains a gel separator and clot activator.
   o Sodium heparin (dark green stopper)
   o Plasma separator tube (PST; light green stopper). Contains lithium heparin anticoagulant and a gel separator.
   o EDTA (lavender stopper)
   o ACDA or ACDB (pale yellow stopper). Contains acid citrate dextrose.
   o Oxalate/fluoride (light gray stopper)

## COMMON ARTERIAL PUNCTURE SITES

The radial artery is the preferred choice for arterial puncture. It is located on the thumb site of the wrist and is most commonly used. The brachial artery is second choice. It is located in the medial anterior aspect of the antecubital area near the biceps tendon insertion. Femoral artery is only used by physicians and trained ER personnel. It is usually used in emergency situations or with patients with low cardiac output.

> **Review Video: Arterial Punctures**
> Visit mometrix.com/academy and enter code: 112543

## APPLYING PRESSURE TO ARTERY AFTER PERFORMING ARTERIAL PUNCTURE

For 3 to 5 minutes directly after the needle is withdrawn from an arterial puncture, a phlebotomist should apply pressure to the puncture site. A patient should not be allowed to hold pressure since they may not hold adequate pressure for the required length of time.

## ULNAR ARTERY

The ulnar artery provides collateral circulation for the hand. Since the radial artery is most commonly used in arterial puncture, the ulnar artery is there as a back up to provide blood to the hand if the radial artery is damaged and becomes unable to supply blood to the hand.

## IF PULSE CANNOT BE FOUND OR IS FAINT AFTER AN ARTERIAL PUNCTURE

If you are unable to find a pulse after an arterial puncture or the pulse is faint, blood flow may be blocked partially or completely by a blood clot. Notify the patient's nurse or physician STAT so that circulation can begin to be restored as quickly as possible.

## ALLEN TEST

The purpose of the Allen test is to determine the presence of collateral circulation in the hand by the ulnar artery.

Allen Test

1. Compress the radial and ulnar arteries with fingers while the patient makes a fist.
2. Patient opens hand; it should have a blanched appearance.
3. The ulnar artery is released and the patient's hand should flush with color. If this occurs, the patient has a positive Allen test and has collateral circulation of the ulnar artery.

## POST CARE OF VENOUS, ARTERIAL, AND CAPILLARY PUNCTURE SITES

**Post care for blood collection sites** include:

- Venous: Place a folded gauze square over puncture site and apply manual pressure for 1 to 2 minutes until bleeding stops (longer if necessary) and then cover with pressure dressing or adhesive bandage.
- Arterial: Place a folded gauze square over the puncture site and apply manual pressure for of 3 to 5 minutes (longer with anticoagulation or coagulopathy). If bleeding, swelling, or bruising persists after initial period of manual pressure, continue pressure for an additional 2 minutes before checking again. The pressure should be maintained until all bleeding has stopped, a pressure bandage should never be used in lieu of manual pressure, and the patient should not apply pressure. Once bleeding stops, clean area with povidone iodine or chlorhexidine and check again in two minutes. Check distal pulse and notify MD if abnormal. Last, apply pressure dressing.
- Capillary: Apply pressure with a clean piece of gauze over the puncture site until bleeding stops. Because the puncture is so small, a bandage is not usually required but can be applied.

## ISSUES THAT AFFECT BLOOD COLLECTION

Many patients have allergies. These include possible allergies to adhesives, latex, and antiseptics. A patient may have a bleeding or bruising disorder that results from a genetic reason or medication that they are taking. Some patients may faint (syncope) during a procedure. It is very appropriate to recline a patient or have the lay down if they have fainted before. Some patients have a fear of needles. Some may experience nausea and vomiting from fear or an illness they have. It may be necessarily to have a trash can or spit-up container nearby for easy access. If a patient his overweight or obese then it may make a collection difficult.

## COMPLICATION OF PHLEBOTOMY

### VASOVAGAL REACTION

A **vasovagal reaction**, characterized by hypotension, diaphoresis, syncope, and nausea, may occur when a patient receives a venipuncture. If a patient complains of feeling faint and appears suddenly pale and shaky during a venipuncture (a vasovagal reaction characterized by diaphoresis and hypotension) the initial response should be to remove the needle because, if the patient faints and falls, it could dislodge the needle and result in trauma. As soon as the needle is removed, sitting patients should be assisted to put their heads low, between their legs. However, the patient is at risk of a fall injury, so the phlebotomist must support the patient. If the patient is in bed, the head of the bed should be lowered. If the patient faints and falls, an incident report must be completed and the patient examined and treated for any injury. The patient may need time to recuperate before another venipuncture is attempted.

### NAUSEA AND VOMITING

Patients may experience **nausea and vomiting** before, during, or after venipuncture because of a nervous response, vasovagal reaction, or current illness. If a patient complains of nausea before the venipuncture begins, the phlebotomist should wait until the symptoms subside unless it is an emergent situation. An emesis basin should be provided for the patient and the patient encouraged to take slow deep breaths to help the person relax. In some cases, applying a cold damp cloth to the patient's forehead may help. If the patient begins to vomit during venipuncture, the procedure should be stopped immediately and a nurse called to assist the patient. The patient should be offered tissues to wipe the mouth and water to rinse the mouth (unless NPO). Some tests may induce nausea in patients, such as the glucose tolerance test.

## CLOTTING DEFICIENCIES, ANTICOAGULANT THERAPY, AND PETECHIAE

Patients with **clotting deficiencies or on anticoagulant therapy**, such as warfarin or heparin, may bleed excessively after venipuncture. Patients are especially at risk for hematomas and persistent bleeding after venipuncture. Steady and prolonged pressure must be applied until bleeding stops. Elevating the arm may help to slow bleeding. A pressure dressing should not be placed instead of maintaining pressure until bleeding stops completely although a pressure dressing may then be applied and left in place for 20-30 minutes after bleeding stops as a precaution. Care must be taken to avoid excessive pressure, which may increase bruising. The phlebotomist should be aware that stroke and heart patients (such as those with atrial fibrillation) often take anticoagulants and should question medications. **Petechiae** may be a sign that a patient has a clotting deficiency, so the phlebotomist should examine the patient's skin carefully and be alert for excessive bleeding after venipuncture.

## NERVE INJURY AND SEIZURES

**Nerve injury** can occur when the needle touches a nerve during a venipuncture, usually the result of poor site selection, improper insertion of needle, or patient movement. The pain is acute, and the patient will generally call out and complain of severe pain, tingling, or "electric shock." The phlebotomist must immediately remove the needle to prevent further damage. Once the bleeding is controlled, an ice pack applied to the site may help to decrease inflammation and pain. The phlebotomist must fill out an incident report and must follow procedures in accordance with facility protocols. Pain may persist for an extended period, and some patients may require physical therapy if nerve damage is severe.

**Seizures** are an uncommon complication and generally unrelated to the venipuncture; however, if a seizure occurs, the phlebotomist should immediately discontinue the venipuncture, apply pressure to the insertion site without restraining the patient and call for help. The phlebotomist should try to prevent the patient from harm. If the patient is seated, the patient may need to be eased onto the floor with assistance.

## EDEMA AND PRIOR MASTECTOMY

Blood should not be drawn from edematous tissue because the **edema** may result in the blood diluted with tissue fluids. Edema is often most pronounced in the hands and feet, but arms may be edematous as well. With generalized edema, the phlebotomist should try to find the least edematous site for venipuncture, should apply gentle pressure to the site to displace the fluid if possible, and should note on the label that edema was present.

Blood generally should not be obtained on the side of a **mastectomy**, regardless of the length of time since surgery, because the circulation may be impaired and edema may be present. Any degree of lymphedema may alter the results of the blood tests, and the patient is at increased risk of infection from venipuncture. If no other site is available, then a physician's order should be obtained regarding use of this site. With double mastectomy, especially if any degree of lymphedema is evident, alternate sites, such as feet and legs may need to be considered. If possible,

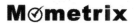

a sample may be obtained through capillary puncture for lymphedema, but for generalized edema, the sample will be diluted.

## PRE-EXISTING INTRAVENOUS LINE

Blood samples should not be obtained from an existing **intravenous line** because the sample may be contaminated with IV fluids/drugs or diluted. Additionally, the sample is more likely to undergo hemolysis and need to be discarded.

Blood should also not be drawn from the same side as an IV line. If blood must be drawn from an arm that has an intravenous line in place, the IV should be clamped for at least two minutes before the specimen is collected to allow the IV fluid to enter the circulation and reduce the dilution of the blood sample. It is preferable to do the venipuncture at least 5 inches distal to the IV insertion site when possible with the tourniquet also applied distal to the IV insertion site. The site (proximal or distal) in relation to the IV should be documented.

## HEMATOMA

During a venipuncture, if the needle goes through the vein and a **hematoma** begins to rapidly develop, the next step is to remove the needle and tourniquet and apply pressure to prevent further loss of blood into the tissue. A hematoma may also form if the needle only partially penetrates the vessel wall, allowing blood to leak into the tissue. If blood flow stops and a small hematoma begins to form, the needle's bevel may be up against a vessel wall, so rotating it slightly may stop the leak and allow blood to flow into the collection tube. If a very small hematoma is evident during venipuncture, the best initial response is to observe the site and complete the venipuncture. If, however, the hematoma is large or expanding, then the phlebotomist should remove the needle, elevate the arm above the level of the heart, and apply pressure until the bleeding stops. Small hematomas are fairly common, especially in older adults whose veins may be friable and those taking anticoagulants and certain other drugs.

## ALLERGIES

Patients should be questioned about **allergies** prior to having blood withdrawn. Common allergies that may pose a problem include:

- <u>Latex:</u> Reactions range from mild to severe anaphylaxis, and latex allergies are increasingly common for those with frequent contact with healthcare, especially those with multiple surgeries and those with spina bifida. The phlebotomist should avoid taking any latex items, such as tourniquets and bandaging supplies, near the patient with a severe allergy and should generally replace latex items with non-latex for all patients.
- <u>Iodine:</u> Patients may be allergic to any skin antiseptic, but allergy to iodine is most common. Patients who report being allergic to fish are also at risk for iodine allergy. Alternate antiseptics should be used in place of antiseptics with iodine.
- <u>Adhesive:</u> Some patients are allergic to adhesive, which may cause itching and rash. Some types of tape, such as paper tape, are better tolerated but may still cause a problem for some patients. Stretch bandaging materials (such as Coban®) may be used to secure a dressing.

## MEDICATIONS AND RECENT SURGERY

**Medications** that pose a particular concern with phlebotomy are those that interfere with clotting mechanisms:

- Platelet inhibitors, such as aspirin, clopidogrel (Plavix®), and abciximab (ReoPro®).
- Anticoagulants include injectable drugs such as heparin, argatroban, and bivalirudin and Oral anticoagulants, such as warfarin (Coumadin®), rivaroxaban (Xarelto®) and Dabigatran (Pradaxa®).

All of these drugs increase the risk of bleeding, so multiple venipunctures should be avoided when possible. Care must be taken to apply pressure until all bleeding stops, and a compression dressing may then be left in place for at least 20 minutes to ensure no recurrence of bleeding.

**Recent surgery** may pose a risk of complications, depending on the type of surgery and the medications given to the patient after surgery. Blood should not be drawn from an arm that has recently undergone any type of surgical procedure or the arm on the side of a mastectomy or any surgery that might interfere with blood flow or lymph flow.

## DEHYDRATION AND CHEMOTHERAPY

**Dehydration** may occur in patients with severe nausea and vomiting and/or diarrhea and those with inadequate fluid intake for body needs. Dehydration results in decreased cardiac output and blood volume, so blood vessels constrict, making it difficult to access the veins and resulting in hemoconcentration that affects test results. If possible, the blood draw should be delayed until the patient is more hydrated; but, if it is necessary to draw blood, a warm compress may help to dilate the vessels slightly. A smaller gauge needle or a winged infusion set may also be necessary. The label should indicate the patient is dehydrated and the physician notified.

Patients on **chemotherapy** often have central lines, such as ports or PICC lines and these may, at times, be used to withdraw samples, but phlebotomists are generally prohibited from drawing specimens through central lines. Veins may be fragile and collapse easily, so a smaller gauge needle or winged infusion set may be necessary. Warming the site may help to make the veins more visible. Edema may obscure veins, and prolonged bleeding may occur because of coagulopathy.

## GERIATRIC ISSUES

Drawing blood from **geriatric patients** poses a number of challenges:

- <u>Disabilities:</u> Patients may be hard of hearing and/or have difficulty speaking, interfering with communication with the patient. The phlebotomist should speak clearly but avoid shouting and allow the patient extra time to respond or indicate comprehension. For patients with vision impairment, the phlebotomist should guide the patient and explain all actions verbally. If a patient has dementia, the phlebotomist should speak in simple sentences and reassure the patient, asking for help if the patient is hostile or combative. Physical disabilities (arthritis, neuromuscular diseases, contractures) may limit mobility.
- <u>Aging:</u> Loose skin and loss of muscle tissue may make it difficult to anchor a vein, and veins may be sclerosed or rolling, so careful anchoring of the vein is necessary. Scarred, sclerosed veins should be avoided. Circulation may be impaired (especially with diabetic patients), and medications (such as anticoagulants) may increase bleeding or interfere with test results. Prolonged pressure may need to be applied to puncture sites, and heavy adhesives may tear skin.

## OBESITY

**Obesity** can pose a problem for venipuncture because the patient's veins may be deep and not visible or palpable. The median cubital vein in the antecubital area should be examined first as it may be palpable between folds of tissue. However, with obese patients, the cephalic vein is often easier to palpate than the median cubital vein. Rotating the hand into prone position (palm down) may make the cephalic vein more palpable. In some cases, a longer needle may be necessary for venipuncture. If there is no or little fat pad on the top of the hand, then the hand veins may be used for venipuncture. Tourniquets may be difficult to position as they tend to roll and twist. An extra-large tourniquet or Velcro closure strap should be used if possible but, if not available, using two tourniquets, one on top of the other, may help keep the tourniquet from twisting. Patients may know from past experience which access site is best, so the phlebotomist should ask the patient directly.

## RISKS TO PATIENTS IF COMPLICATIONS OR ERRORS OCCUR IN BLOOD COLLECTION

The following are some of the risks to patients if a complication or error results from blood collection:

1. Arterial puncture
2. Anemia resulting from the procedure
3. Infection
4. Hematoma (bruising) of the venipuncture site
5. Damage to a nerve if punctured
6. Vein damage
7. Pain

## HEMATOMA

Described below is how a hematoma can result from errors in phlebotomy techniques:

1. inadequate pressure to the collection site after a blood draw
2. blood leaking through the back of a vein that was pierced
3. blood leaking from a partial pierced vein
4. an artery is pierced

# EDTA

**Ethylenediaminetetraacetic acid (EDTA)** is a potassium-based or sodium-based anticoagulant used in blood collection tubes (usually lavender and pink) to prevent clotting of the whole blood specimens (CBC and blood component tests) and to save specimens for blood bank testing. EDTA binds calcium to prevent clotting and preserves cell morphology and prevents the aggregation of platelets. The tube should be filled to the specified level and the correct tube size selected for the necessary volume. Eight to 10 inversions are needed immediately after sample collection in order to thoroughly mix EDTA with the blood because failure to adequately mix them can result in formation of microclots or aggregated platelets. EDTA may be in liquid form (K3EDTA) or spray-dried (K2EDTA), but the liquid form may dilute the sample and alter test results (1-2% decrease). EDTA tube with blood sample should be placed in a refrigerator while awaiting processing. The timing and storage requirements vary according to the type of test. For example, red blood cells count remains stable for up to 72 hours under refrigeration, but white blood cell counts are less stable.

## ETHANOL (BLOOD ALCOHOL) TEST

**Ethanol** (ETHOH), commonly referred to as "blood alcohol", tests may be done for clinical or legal reasons. If carried out for legal reasons, such as to determine if a driver was under the influence of alcohol, chain of custody protocols must be followed and carefully documented. Special considerations:

- Skin antiseptics containing alcohol (isopropyl alcohol, methanol, tincture of iodine) cannot be used because they may contaminate the specimen and alter test results. Alternate skin antiseptics include povidone-iodine and aqueous benzalkonium chloride. If no alternative is available, the site should be thoroughly washed with soap and water and dried.
- Alcohol readily evaporates, so the collection tube should be completely filled and the stopper should be left on the tube until ready to perform testing.
- Testing may be done on whole blood, serum, or plasma. A glass grey top, sodium fluoride tube, with or without anticoagulant, is usually used.

## TERMS

**Malpractice**: A lawsuit raised against a professional for injury or loss resulting from negligence on the part of the professional in rendering services.

**Negligence**: Failure to perform or act with the prudence expected by a reasonable person in the same circumstance.

**DNR**: Do not resuscitate. No codes should be called for this patient and no heroic measures should be taken to revive patient if the patient stops breathing.

**NPO**: From the Latin phrase nil per os meaning nothing by mouth. Patients are not allowed food or drink including water. This restriction is usually placed on a patient before and after a procedure.

**STAT**: From the Latin word statim means immediately. It describes the need for a specimen or test to be done immediately in response to critical situations with the possibility of the test results preventing a patient's death.

**ASAP**: As soon as possible, this is used if the results are needed soon but not to prevent the patient from dying

**Fasting**: When a person refrains from eating or drinking anything before a procedure, sometimes water is allowed on a fast

**Bevel**: Slanted tip of a needle used to puncture the skin and vein without removing a piece of the vein.

**Plunger**: The part of the syringe that when pulled on creates a vacuum allowing the barrel of the syringe to be filled with fluid or air.

**Hub**: End of a needle that attaches to the blood collection device i.e. syringe or tube holder

**Shaft**: The hollow round long cylinder-shaped part of a needle

**Sharps container**: An easily sealed, rigid, leak-proof, puncture-resistant, disposable box with a locking lid in which used needles and sharp materials are disposed.

## TRUE OR FALSE QUESTIONS

Determine if each of the following is true or false:

1. A typical blood donor unit contains 450 mL of blood.
2. A paternity test can prove that a specific child has been fathered by a specific male.
3. Eating sugarless foods cannot affect the results of a glucose tolerance test.
4. Turnaround time in a lab refers to the time between the drawing of testing specimen and the return of the testing results.
5. Adhesive bandages should not be used on children younger than 2.
6. OSHA does not require that sharps containers be labeled with a biohazard symbol.
7. A 1:10 dilution of 5.25% sodium hypochlorite is effective in killing HIV when used as a disinfectant
8. Butterfly needles are the standard needles used for routine venipuncture.
9. An arteriospasm occurs when improper technique is used.
10. Arterial puncture is extremely painful.
11. Vasovagal syncope is due to large amounts of blood being draw.
12. The best way to tell if a specimen is arterial is by its color.

## ANSWERS

1. A typical blood donor unit contains 450 mL of blood. **True**
2. False: A paternity test can prove without a doubt that that a specific child has been fathered by a specific male. **False**, a paternity test cannot prove with complete certainty that a specific male has fathered a specific child. It can however prove that a specific male did NOT father a specific child.
3. Eating sugarless foods cannot affect the results of a glucose tolerance test. **False**, sugarless foods can affect the digestive process, and this can in turn affect the glucose tolerance test results.
4. Turnaround time in a lab refers to the time between the drawing of testing specimen and the return of the testing results. **False**, turnaround time starts when the order is received not when the draw of the testing specimen is completed.
5. **True**, adhesive bandages pose a choking hazard to children under the age of two.
6. **False**, OSHA requires all sharps containers to be marked with a biohazard symbol
7. **True**, also known as household bleach, this solution has been proven to kill HIV as well as HBV.
8. **False**, butterfly needles are used with infants and with difficult veins. 21-gauge needle is the standard needle used for routine venipuncture.
9. An arteriospasm can occur when proper technique is used. It is a reflexive constricting of the artery, possibly caused by anxiety, pain, or arterial muscle irritation. **False**
10. Arterial puncture is more painful than venipuncture, but it should not be extremely painful. Extreme pain indicates that a nerve has been involved in the procedure, and the procedure should stop. **False**
11. Vasovagal syncope is due hypotension as the result of abrupt pain or trauma. **False**
12. The best way to tell if a specimen is arterial is by the way the blood pumps into the syringe. **False**

# Special Collections

### ACCEPTABLE BLOOD SMEAR

A blood smear will be spread over one-half to three-fourths of the slide. There will be a gradual shift from thick to thin blood smear on the slide with the thinnest part of the slide being one blood cell thick. This thinnest part of the blood smear is sometimes referred to as the "feather." The feather part of the blood smear is the most important since the differential is performed there. In blood smears made using the two-slide method hold the slide that will smear the blood droplet at a 30-degree angle to the slide that the blood droplet was placed on.

### AEROBIC AND ANAEROBIC COLLECTION

Blood collection for **blood cultures** usually involves collecting samples in two containers:

- Aerobic container: Contains air and medium to encourage growth of aerobic organisms.
- Anaerobic container: Is a vacuum and contains no air but contains a medium to encourage growth of anaerobic organisms.

Blood cultures may be done to determine the cause of fever of unknown origin and to determine if bacteremia is present. If a needle and syringe is used to collect the specimen, the anaerobic container is filled first and then the aerobic container. If a winged infusion set ("butterfly) is used, then the aerobic bottle is filled first because the tubing may contain a small amount of air. If multiple sets are ordered at the same time, each set must be obtained from a separate site although waiting 30 minutes between obtaining specimens is recommended.

### NEWBORN SCREENING

While the March of Dimes recommends **newborn screening** for 31 disorders, including hearing deficit, the list of screened diseases varies somewhat, and some states include infectious diseases, such as HIV and toxoplasmosis. All states require testing for PKU, galactosemia, and hypothyroidism, and 44 states and the District of Colombia require at least 29 of the 31 recommended tests. The blood sample should be obtained between 24 and 72 hours after birth because earlier testing may be inaccurate for some disorders, so repeat testing in 2 weeks is required in some states. Tests are carried out through blood spot collection with a heel puncture. The first drop of blood is wiped away, and then a large drop is placed in the center of each circle, being careful to avoid double drops, which may interfere with results, and to fill the circles and penetrate the paper without touching the circles with the child's foot or with the gloved hand. The spot collection papers should be placed horizontally to dry but should not be stacked or hung before or after drying.

### COLLECTION OF STOOL SPECIMENS

**Stool specimens** are obtained by placing a stool collection device in a toilet or in a bedpan. The specimen is then placed in a clean specimen container, or if for cultures, in a sterile container. Different types of containers may be used, with or without preservatives, depending on the type of tests being conducted. The sample is transferred using a tongue blade to the fill-line indicated on the container. If an additive is in the container, the sample should be shaken to mix contents. The container should be properly labeled and sealed in a biohazard bag for transport. For a stool culture, the specimen should be collected before the patient begins antibiotics. The stool specimen is placed in a sterile container or a cotton-tipped swab is inserted into the rectum and rotated to

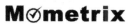

obtain a fecal sample. Then the swab is inserted into a sterile tube. Stools specimens should be processed as soon as possible or stored at 4° C if delay of more than two hours before processing.

## COLLECTION AND PRESERVATION OF EXTRAVASCULAR BODY FLUIDS FOR CHEMICAL ANALYSIS

| | |
|---|---|
| **Amniotic fluid** | Sample collected by a physician during amniocentesis. Store in special container (protected from light) at room temperature for chromosome analysis or on ice for some chemistry tests (according to protocol). |
| **Cerebrospinal fluid** | Sample collected by physician. Collect in 3 tubes (first for culture and others for chemistry and microscopy) and store at room temperature with immediate delivery to lab. *Neisseria meningitidis* is fragile and cold sensitive, so do not chill specimen. |
| **Gastric fluids** | Sample collected during gastroscopy or from NG tube. Store in sterile container at room temperature for up to 6 hours, refrigerated for up to 7 days and frozen for up to 30 days. |
| **Nasopharyngeal secretions.** | Collected with swab or nasopharyngeal area. Place swab in tube with transport medium. |
| **Saliva** | Collected in sterile container after patient rinses mouth and waits a few minutes. Test immediately (point of care) or freeze for hormone tests to maintain stability. |
| **Semen** | Collect fresh sample from individual immediately following ejaculation into sterile container. Keep sample warm and deliver immediately for testing. |
| **Serous fluid** | Sample collected by physician, typically through thoracentesis or paracentesis. Samples labeled as pleural, peritoneal, or pericardial. Place in sterile container for C&S, EDTA tube for cell counts/smears, oxalate or fluoride tubes for chemistry tests. |
| **Synovial fluid** | Sample collected by physician through aspiration of joint. Place in ETDA or heparin tube for cell counts, smear, and crystal identification; sterile tube for C&S; and plain tube for chemistry and immunology tests. |
| **Sputum** | First morning production of sputum preferred because a larger volume is likely to be produced after sleeping. Patients should remove any dentures and rinse mouth before attempting to cough up specimen. Transport at room temperature and process immediately. |
| **Urine** | Collected in sterile container form midstream urination or catheterization. If for 24-hour quantitative testing, urine is collected in a 2L container. Store at room temperature in sterile container for 2 hours (protected from light) and then refrigerate. If both UA and C&S required, then test or refrigerate immediately. |

## NONBLOOD FLUID SPECIMENS

Listed below are several nonblood fluid specimens routinely collected for analysis from the human body:

1. 1.Urine
2. Amniotic Fluid
3. Cerebrospinal Fluid
4. Gastric Secretions
5. Nasopharyngeal Secretions

6. Saliva
7. Semen
8. Serous Fluids
9. Sputum
10. Sweat
11. Synovial Fluid

## AFP

AFP is alpha-fetoprotein. Normally it is found in the human fetus, but abnormal levels of AFP may indicate a neural tube defect in an infant or other fetal developmental problems. The test is performed on maternal serum. If results are abnormal, a test on the amniotic fluid will be used to confirm results.

## URINE TESTS

The following are some common urine tests:

1. Routine Urinalysis
2. Culture and Sensitivity – diagnosis urinary tract infection
3. Cytology Studies – presence of abnormal cells from urinary tract
4. Drug Screening – detects illegal use of drugs (prescription or illicit) and steroid, also monitors therapeutic drug use.
5. Pregnancy Test – confirms pregnancy by testing for the presence of HCG

## 24-HOUR URINE SPECIMEN COLLECTION

All urine must be collected over the course of 24 hours. A large collection container is given to the patient. When a patient awakes, the first void of the morning is for the previous 24 hours and must be discarded. The next void is collected as well as the next void over the next 24 hours as well as the next morning void. Sometimes the specimen collection has to be refrigerated.

## MIDSTREAM URINE COLLECTION AND MIDSTREAM CLEAN-CATCH URINE COLLECTION

Both involve and initial void into the toilet, interruption of urine flow, the restart of urination into a collection container, collection of a sufficient amount of specimen, and voiding of excess urine down the toilet. The clean-catch involves cleaning of the genital area, collecting urine into a sterile container and quick processing to prevent overgrowth of microorganisms, degradation of the specimen, and incorrect results.

## ASPECTS OF URINE REVIEWED IN URINALYSIS

The following aspects of urine are reviewed in a routine urinalysis:

- Physical- color, odor, transparency, specific gravity
- Chemical- looking for bacteria, blood, WBC, protein, and glucose
- Microscopic – urine components i.e. casts, cells, and crystals

## TERMS

**Blood smear**: blood layer on a glass slide made from a drop of blood

**Capillary blood gases**: blood gases retrieved from an arterialized skin puncture

**Interstitial fluid**: liquid found between cells

**Intracellular fluid**: liquid found within cell membranes

# Processing

## ALIQUOT

When a specimen is collected, it may need to be divided to run several tests on it. An aliquot is a fraction of the specimen. Each aliquot has its own tube for testing and is label with the same information as the original specimen.

## ELECTROLYTE ANALYSIS

Bicarbonate, chloride, potassium and sodium are the four most commonly tested for electrolytes.

## ANALYTES THAT BREAK DOWN IN LIGHT

The following are some commonly tested for analytes that can be broken down in the presence of light:

- Bilirubin
- Vitamin $B_{12}$
- Urine Porphyrins

## REASONS SPECIMENS MAY BE REJECTED FOR ANALYSIS

Some reasons why a specimen may be rejected for testing include incorrect or incomplete identification, collected in an expired tube, inadequate amount of specimen collected (QNS, quantity not sufficient), and collection in an incorrect tube.

## MINIMUM REQUIREMENTS FOR LABELING SPECIMENS

Laboratory specimens should always be **labeled** after collection with a label that is permanently attached (with adhesive). The tube or other container should never be labeled in advance, and permanent ink (generally black) should be used for any lettering:

- No pre-printed label: A label must be hand-lettered with required information, which must include the patient's full name, ID number (temporary or permanent) if available, date of birth, date and time of specimen collection, and the phlebotomist's signature or initials.
- Pre-printed label: If a label is preprinted with the patient's name and other identifying information and/or a barcode, the phlebotomist must attach the label and write the date and time on the letter and sign with signature or initials.

Any special considerations, such as "fasting" should be noted on the label as well. Before the phlebotomist leaves the patient's side, the phlebotomist should compare the label on the specimen to the patient's ID bracelet or record and the laboratory requisition to ensure they all match. Once labeled, the specimen should be placed in a biohazard bag or container for transport.

## IMPORTANCE OF PROPER HANDLING OF SPECIMEN BEFORE ANALYSIS

46 to 68% of lab errors result from improper handling of a specimen before it was analyzed. For example, if an anticoagulant tube is improperly mixed, it may result in microclots forming. If a tube is shaken too hard hemolysis of the specimen may occur. If a specimen is not cooled properly then metabolic processes may continue after collection which may skew test results.

## CHAIN-OF-CUSTODY SPECIMENS

**Chain-of-custom specimens** are those for which a laboratory has established a documented record that shows every consecutive person in contact with the specimen from the time of collection through transfer and to the time of disposition (both internal and external contact and including date, time, and signature) and ensures that no tampering with the specimen has occurred in order to meet legal requirements. The document must outline provisions for securing long-term storage. Chain-of-custom specimens may include specimens for blood alcohol, drugs, or crime scene testing, often including blood, urine and DNA testing. The chain-of-custom SOP may include labeling requirements, temperature requirements, expected timeline, packing, and transporting specifications. The person from whom the sample is obtained must be clearly identified as well as the name of the collector and the time, date, and location of obtaining the sample. Containers in which a sample is transported should be secured with custody tape.

## INTERPERSONAL COMMUNICATION WITH NON-LABORATORY PERSONNEL

**Interpersonal communication** skills are essential for the laboratory professional, who must interact with a variety of non-laboratory personnel in the work environment. Elements of effective communication include:

- Showing respect and consideration to others in all communications.
- Recognizing each individual's scope of practice and responsibilities toward the patient.
- Being an active listener, paying attention and asking clarifying questions as necessary.
- Sharing important information with the appropriate personnel.
- Asking questions when in need of more information about a patient.
- Ensuring that information is shared accurately.
- Providing timely communication.
- Discussing special needs of patients in relation to collection of a sample and processing.
- Communicating any problems encountered with collection or processing with the appropriate personnel.
- Discussing timing issues related to sample collection, such as STAT orders or collection that must be done at a specific time.
- Scheduling collection to avoid interrupting other patient care activities when possible.

## SPECIMEN ASSESSMENT AND REJECTION CRITERIA

Specimens must be obtained following established protocols and in the proper tube or container with the correct additive, such as sodium citrate in a blood specimen. The specimen must be stored and/or transported in a manner appropriate to the type of specimen. **Rejection criteria** may vary according to the type of specimen and test, and specimens are generally not discarded until the ordering healthcare provider is notified. Rejection criteria may include:

- Incorrect tube or container.
- Incorrect or missing requisition/order.
- Specimen size insufficient for testing.
- Hemolysis evident.
- Specimen not correctly labeled.
- Tube/container leaking or contaminated with body fluids. (Note: critical specimens may be salvaged after tube/container thoroughly cleansed with 10% hypochlorite [bleach] solution.)
- Specimen contained in syringe with attached needle.
- Date/Collection time not noted on specimen.

- Specimen too old for testing.
- Specimen improperly stored/transported.

## LABORATORY RESULTS

Information that must be included on the **laboratory results** includes the name, address, and contact information for the lab, the patient's name, birthdate, gender, and ID number (if one is assigned) and the name of the requesting provider. The results must include the date and time the specimen was collected and the date and time each test result was verified. The tests should be listed along with the value, units, and reference ranges with some indication of abnormal values, such a high (H) or low (L), abnormal (A), critical high (CH) or critical low (CL). The lab results should be separated by type, such as chemistry panels and hematology panels. Laboratory results may be distributed to ordering providers in a number of different ways:

- Paper: May be delivered by courier, placed in physician's hospital mailbox, or mailed.
- Telephone: Results may be transmitted by phone even when paper or other type of report is given to ensure that the ordering provider receives the information in a timely manner, especially when there are abnormal results.
- Messaging/Email/Electronic: Must be delivered over secure lines so that confidentiality is not compromised. Reports may be sent automatically. If patients can access through a patient portal, the ordering provider may need to access the report first and indicate it can be released to the patient, depending on how the system is set up.

## ASSESSING SPECIMEN QUALITY

Issues of **specimen quality** include:

- Hemolysis: Pink discoloration of plasma and serum because of the presence of damaged red blood cells and hemoglobin. May result from abnormal condition, such as hemolytic anemia, or from incorrect handling. Hemolyzed samples may interfere with some tests (electrolytes, iron, enzymes), so the sample will likely need to be redrawn.
- Quantity not sufficient (QNS): May occur if the volume of blood in the collection tube is insufficient for testing or if the blood-anticoagulant ratio is incorrect. Short draws may be sufficient for some tests if the specimen is not hemolyzed. With QNS, the usual solution is to obtain another specimen.
- Clotting: May result from maintaining a sample in a syringe with no anticoagulant for too long before transferring to a tube, carrying out a very slow draw with a syringe that allows clotting to begin, and failing to adequately mix the sample with the anticoagulant. If clotting occurs, a new sample must be obtained.
- Incorrect specimen type: If the incorrect specimen type is obtained or a specimen is obtained in a collection tube with the wrong additive, then another specimen must be obtained in order to carry out the intended tests.

## ALIQUOTING

**Aliquoting** a sample is done to withdraw serum or plasma from whole blood and/or to divide one sample into multiple aliquots for different tests. The individual must apply PPI, including gloves and goggles, and prepare aliquot tubes with appropriate labels. Aliquoting is done after centrifugation with anticoagulated tubes aliquoted into plasma specimens and coagulated tube aliquoted into serum specimens. It's necessary to place the centrifuged tubes into a rack and to avoid inverting the sample after centrifugation because this will cause remixing. A disposable pipette (never use a mouth pipette) is used to transfer each aliquot, starting from the top of the sample and working downward toward the point of separation. The aliquots are transferred to labeled tubes. As soon as an aliquot tube is filled, it must be capped. Aliquoted samples must be carefully labeled because serum and plasma are indistinguishable once they are aliquoted. Some other types of samples, such as saliva, must be mixed using a vortex mixer prior to aliquoting to ensure the sample is homogenous. Aliquots should be placed promptly in the appropriate storage, such as the refrigerator or -20° or -80° C freezer.

## SETTLING OF BLOOD IN ANTICOAGULANT TUBES

Described below is how blood in an anticoagulant tube will settle after being centrifuged or being allowed to settle:

- The top layer will be the plasma.
- The next thin layer is the buffy coat made of white blood cells and platelets.
- The bottom layer is red blood cells.

## PROPERLY CENTRIFUGING A SPECIMEN

The centrifuge needs to be evenly balanced with tubes of equal size and volume across from one another. Stoppers should always be in place to prevent aerosol. Also, be sure to allow complete clotting before centrifuging the specimen. If a specimen is not completely clotted before centrifuging then it may result in latent fibrin formations clotting the serum. Never centrifuge a specimen twice.

## CHILLING A SPECIMEN

The most appropriate way to chill a specimen is to immerse it into an ice and water slush. Ice cubes alone will not allow for adequate cooling of the specimen, and where the ice cubes touch the specimen may freeze it resulting in possible hemolysis or breakdown of the analyte.

## INVERTING A TUBE

A tube should be inverted if it contains an additive and if the manufacturer's instructions require for it to be inverted. If the tube in a nonadditive tube then it does not have to be inverted. An additive tube usually is inverted between three and eight times to properly mix the additive with the blood.

## PREVENTING AEROSOL FORMATION WHEN STOPPER HAS NO SAFETY FEATURE TO PREVENT AEROSOL

The stopper should be covered with 4x4-inch gauze and placed behind a safety shield to ensure the aerosol is not inhaled. Proper protective clothing should be worn as well. A safety stopper removal device may also be used.

## TEMPERATURE REQUIREMENTS FOR SPECIMENS

Specimen storage is often at room **temperature**, which is generally based on the range found in temperature-controlled buildings: 20° C to 25° C. Blood bank and laboratory specimen refrigerators are maintained between 2° C and 4° C. Freezers are maintained at -20° C with some specialty freezers at -80° C. Incubators usually provide for a range of temperatures (5° C to 70° C) with much incubation done at 37° C (body temperature). Samples may remain viable for different periods of time, depending on how they are stored. Some serum and plasma samples must be frozen prior to shipping. Temperature requirements depend on the types of specimen and the test.

| Transport with heat block at 37° C | Transport in ice slurry and refrigerate (freezing may cause hemolysis) |
|---|---|
| Cryoglobulins, cryofibrinogen, and cold agglutinin. | ACTH, acetone, ACE, ammonia, blood gases, catecholamines, FFA, gastrin, glucagon, homocysteine, lactic acid, PTH, blood pH, pyruvate, renin. |

## SHIPPING PATIENT SAMPLES

Note that personnel responsible for **shipping** of specimens must have been appropriately trained and understand possible hazards, according to regulations by the Department of Transportation, International Civil Aviation Organization, and CDC. Frozen serum and plasma must be shipped in plastic tubes (not glass) with screw-on caps for security and labeled with 2 patient identifiers. The tubes are wrapped in absorbent material in case of leakage and secured in a container that is airtight (such as Saf-T-Pak®) and labeled "biohazard," placed inside of a Styrofoam container for insulation with dry ice and in a clearly labeled secure box or in a temperature- controlled container. Specimens that are not frozen are similarly packaged: specimen container, wrapped in absorbent material and placed in individual biohazard bag and secured in transport box of metal or plastic. The specimen may or may not be placed in a temperature-controlled container, depending on ambient temperatures.

## LIGHT CONSIDERATIONS IN TRANSPORTING SPECIMENS AND DISPOSITION OF SPECIMENS

Most specimens are not sensitive to **light**, but some must be transported in special light-blocking containers or wrapped in aluminum foil during transport: bilirubin, carotene, red cell folate, serum folate, vitamin B2, 6, and 12, and vitamin C. Urine specimens for porphyrins and porphobilinogen must also be protected from light. Light-blocking amber colored collection tubes and urine specimen containers are also available OSHA and state regulations outline the requirements for **disposition** of blood bags and patient samples. Blood disposition must comply with OSHA's Bloodborne Pathogen's Standard (29 CFR 1910.1030), which covers blood (semi-liquid, liquid, dried) in containers, in other waste products, or on items, such as sharps. As a regulated waste, the blood must be placed in a container that is closable, leak-proof, labeled (proper color-coding), and closed before removal to avoid any spillage or loss of contents during transport to disposal site.

## TIME CONSIDERATIONS WHEN PROCESSING SAMPLES

Specimens should be delivered to the laboratory for processing as quickly as possible and within no more than 45 minutes. Stat tests should be run first. Some tests have **time considerations** that must be followed:

- Blood gases must be processed within 20 minutes.
- Prothrombin time (PT) must be run on unrefrigerated blood sample within 24 hours.
- Partial thromboplastin time (PTT) must be run on room temperature or refrigerated sample within 4 hours.

Additives also affect time considerations:

| Additive | Tests | Time from collection |
|---|---|---|
| EDTA | Blood smear | Within one hour. |
| ETDA | CBC | Within 6 hours at room temperature; within 4 hours for micro-collection tubes. However, sample usually stable at room temperature for 24 hours. |
| EDTA | ESR | With 4 hours at room temperature; within 12 hours if refrigerated. |
| EDTA | Reticulocyte count | Within 6 hours at room temperature and 72 hours if refrigerated. |
| Sodium fluoride | Glucose | Within 24 hours at room temperature and 48 hours if refrigerated. |

## PROCEDURES TO PREVENT HEMOLYSIS

**Hemolysis**, rupture of red blood cells, is the most common reason laboratory specimens must be redrawn. Steps to preventing hemolysis include:

1. Utilize large gauge (20 to 22) needle for blood draws for large veins, such as the antecubital.
2. Warm draw site to improve blood flow.
3. Keep tourniquet on no longer than 60 seconds.
4. Air-dry alcohol applied to skin prior to blood draw.
5. Utilize partial vacuum tubes if possible.
6. Avoid milking veins or capillary puncture sites.
7. Avoid excessive pressure when pulling or pushing on plunger.
8. Avoid blood draws from catheters or vascular access devices.
9. Ensure volume in tubes with anticoagulant is sufficient.
10. Avoid vigorous mixing or shaking of specimens.
11. Invert tubes with clot activator 5 times, with anticoagulant 8 to 10 times, and with sodium citrate 3 to 4 times (coagulation tests).
12. Store and transport specimens at appropriate temperature.
13. Use appropriate centrifugal speed and duration for processing samples that have clotted completely.

## BLOOD CULTURE PROCESS

The general blood culture collection is as follows:

- Verify patient identification with two identifiers.
- Use standard precautions and venipuncture procedures, and use aseptic technique when handling equipment to avoid contamination.
- Vigorously scrub skin with antiseptic for 30 to 60 seconds to remove skin bacteria and allow to dry.
- Swab caps of blood culture bottles with antiseptic. Note fill line.
- Carry out blood draw. Adults: 10-20 mL per set and pediatric patients 1-2 mL per set.
- If multiple draws are ordered, wait 30 minutes between draws unless otherwise ordered. Take multiple draws from different sites.
- Replace venipuncture needle with blunt fill needle and use transfer device.
- Inject blood culture specimen into both anaerobic and aerobic bottles.
- Mix specimen with medium in the culture bottle according to directions.

- Label culture bottles.
- Dispose of contaminated equipment and sharps in appropriate containers.
- Remove gloves, sanitize hands, and transport specimen to the laboratory. Incubate and monitor as per protocol.

## CLOTTING TIME

**Clotting time** may vary according to environmental conditions and addition of clot activators. Clotting must be fully complete before a sample is placed in the centrifuge or latent formation of fibrin may clot serum. Complete clotting usually takes between 30 and 60 minutes at temperatures of 22 to 25° C (room temperature) although this time may be prolonged in samples with a high white blood cell count or in chilled samples. Clotting is also prolonged in samples of patients on anticoagulant therapy, such as heparin or warfarin. Clot activators may be added to a sample to decrease the time needed for clotting:

1. Silica particles (found in serum separator tubes) and plastic red-topped tubes require 15 to 30 minutes.
2. Thrombin tubes require about 5 minutes.

Note: 5 to 6 gentle inversions of tubes with clot activators to mix it with the blood sample are required.

## COMPUTER-GENERATED LABEL

The label would contain the patient's name, date of birth or age, medical record number, collection time (in military time).

## RAM AND ROM

RAM is temporary computer data storage. RAM stands for Random Access Memory. If RAM is not saved into a permanent file the information will be lost if the computer is turned off.

ROM is read-only memory. ROM is memory whose contents can be accessed and read but cannot be easily changed. When a computer is turned off and turned back on the ROM has not changed.

## PURPOSE OF A PASSWORD

A password is unique to each computer user. It should be kept confidential. A password allows access to a computer and identifies who the computer user is when used in conjunction with an ID code. When the ID code or password is used to obtain access to a computer, this is called logging on.

## LIS

An LIS is a laboratory information system. Usually the LIS is used to order tests, print labels for specimens, and enter test results. LIS can be customized to specific laboratory requirements.

## SAMPLE REGISTRATION

**Sample registration** begins with patient registration, which enters identifying information about the patient into the system. If an electronic laboratory information system (LIS) is in use, then labels and barcodes for specimen tubes are generated during patient registration. When the specimen is brought to the laboratory for processing, the sample is registered as part of the existing patient registration by retrieving the patient's file, based on ID number assigned during registration and inputting information. If a LIS is not in use and laboratory records are done manually, labels and barcodes may be generated on arrival at the lab. The sample is assigned a number and the time of the collection noted as well as arrival time and the type of tube and additive. Location tracking

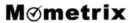

begins, with the record indicating exactly where the sample is placed, such as the shelf, container, row, and number in a refrigerator if the sample is stored.

## INTERNAL AND EXTERNAL DATABASES

A **database** is a computerized collection of files and stored data. Most databases used in healthcare are relational databases, which are built on a multiple table structure with each individual item on a table having a unique identifier. Data found in a database can be accessed through queries, updated, deleted, or revised. Internal databases are maintained within an organization and are often used for patient registration information, budget, and inventory. External databases, on the other hand, are contained in servers outside of the organization (sometimes in the cloud). The data found in an internal database may be backed up in an external database in a remote server for security reasons. An external database may be accessed with proper authority, and data may be linked to that in the internal database so it is easily accessible. In some cases, data from an external database can be imported directly into the internal database.

## HEPARIN

The purpose of heparin is to prevent coagulation. The three types of heparin are ammonium, sodium and lithium. Ammonium heparin is used for hematocrit determinations and is found in capillary tubes. Sodium heparin and lithium heparin are used in evacuated tubes. Just be sure that the heparin that is being used is not what is being tested. For example, heparin is used for electrolyte testing, but sodium is a commonly tested electrolyte thus sodium heparin would not be an appropriate heparin to use to test for electrolytes. It is important to mix heparin tubes properly to prevent microclots.

## TRACE AND ULTRATRACE ELEMENTS

**Trace elements** are metals and may include iron, lead, zinc, mercury, aluminum, and copper. **Ultratrace elements** include boron, nickel, vanadium, arsenic and silicon. Specimens may easily be contaminated so care must be taken to avoid any specimen containers with metal. Special trace-element-free specimen tubes (usually royal blue and containing EDTA, heparin, or no additive) should be used because trace metals may be found in standard glass and plastic tubes and in the stoppers. Because some substances—gadolinium, iodine, and barium contrast—interfere with test results, testing should be delayed for at least 96 hours if patients have received any of these. The specimens must be kept clean and protected from dust. No iodine products should be used for antisepsis, only alcohol. When transferring plasma or serum, it must be poured into aliquots and not transferred by a pipette. Labels are color-coded to indicate the type of additive: lavender indicates EDTA; green, heparin; and red, no additive.

## TERMS

**Accession Number**: Unique number given for each test request

**Aerosol**: Substance released in the form of a fine mist

**Barcode**: Series of black bars and white spaces spaced at intentional, unique distances to represent numbers and letters

**Centrifugation**: The process of substance separation by spinning

**Impermeable**: Does not allow the passage of liquids

**CPU**: Central Processing Unit, the command center of the computer

**Cursor**: Blinking marker on the computer screen that indicates where information should be inputted

**Hardware**: The mechanical, magnetic, electronic, and electrical components making up a computer system

**Interface**: A connection between hardware devices, applications, or different sections of a computer network

**Monitor**: A device similar to a television screen that receives video signals from the computer and displays the information for the user

## TRUE OR FALSE QUESTIONS

Determine if each of the following is true or false:

1. Wrapping a specimen in aluminum foil is a good way to protect it from light.
2. According to NCCLS guidelines, a specimen should be separated ASAP with 2 hours being the absolute time limit.
3. A cold agglutinin requires special transportation at body temperature.
4. If unfamiliar with a requested test, a phlebotomist should refer to the laboratory user manual for information and instructions about the test.

## ANSWERS

1. Wrapping a specimen in aluminum foil is a good way to protect it from light. **True**
2. According to NCCLS guidelines, a specimen should be separated ASAP with 2 hours being the absolute time limit. **True**
3. A cold agglutinin requires special transportation at body temperature. **True**
4. If unfamiliar with a requested test, a phlebotomist should refer to the laboratory user manual for information and instructions about the test. **True**

# Core Knowledge

## ANEMIA

Anemia refers to any condition where there is reduced oxygen carrying capacity due to a fall in hemoglobin concentration with resultant tissue hypoxia. It is defined as Hb less than 13.5g/dl in males, <11/5g/dl in females, <15g/dl in newborns to three-month-olds, and less than 11g/dl from three months to puberty. Anemia results when compensatory mechanisms fail to restore oxygen levels to meet tissue demands. The following compensatory mechanisms are seen – arteriolar dilatation, increased cardiac output, increased anaerobic metabolism, increased Hb dissociation, increased erythropoietin output, and internal redistribution of blood flow. If these compensatory mechanisms are adequate, oxygen levels are restored. If not, anemia ensues, with cardiac effects, poor exercise tolerance, lethargy, pallor, headaches, angina on effort, and claudication.

## LAYERS OF THE HEART

Three layers of tissue form the heart wall. The outer layer of the heart wall is the epicardium, the middle layer is the myocardium, and the inner layer is the endocardium:

- Epicardium- the membrane that covers the outside of the heart
- Myocardium-The muscular wall of the heart, the thickest of the three layers of the heart wall, it lies between the inner layer (endocardium) and the outer layer (epicardium).
- Endocardium- membrane lining the inside surface of heart

## HEART CHAMBERS AND VALVES

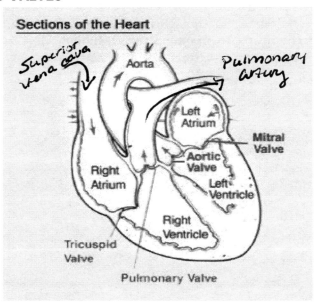

## CARDIAC CYCLE

Ventricular Systole:

1. ventricles contract
2. ventricular contraction regulated by AV node
3. semilunar valves (to aorta & pulmonary arteries) open
4. atrioventricular valves close ("lub")

Ventricular Diastole:

1. ventricles relax, atria contract
2. atrial contraction regulated by SA node (pacemaker)
3. semilunar valves close ("dupp")
4. atrioventricular valves open

## ORIGIN OF HEART SOUNDS

A single heartbeat lasts about one second and consists of a two-part pumping action. As blood collects in both atria (the upper chambers of the heart), the SA node (the heart's natural pacemaker) sends an electrical signal that causes atrial contraction. This contraction forces blood through the mitral and tricuspid valves into the resting ventricles (the lower chambers). This is the longer part of the two-part pumping phase, and it is termed diastole. The pumping phase's second part begins when the ventricles have filled with blood. The electrical impulses from the SA node reach the AV node and then travel to the ventricles, signaling them to contract. This phase is called systole. During ventricular contraction, the mitral and tricuspid valves close tightly to prevent the back flow of blood, but the aortic and pulmonary valves are forced open. Blood ejected from the right ventricle travels to the lungs to get oxygenated. Oxygen-rich blood leaves the left ventricle to travel to all other areas of the body. The ventricles relax, and the pulmonary and aortic valves close after blood enters the aorta and pulmonary artery. The lower pressure in the ventricles causes the tricuspid and mitral valves to open, and the cycle begins again. This system of contractions is repeated, increasing during times of exertion and decreasing while at rest.

## ELECTRICAL CONDUCTION SYSTEM

The heart beats (contracts) as a result of electrical impulses from the heart muscle (the myocardium). The electrical impulse starts in the sinoatrial node (SA node), which is located in the top of the right atrium. Sometimes the SA node is referred to as the heart's "natural pacemaker." When the SA node releases the electrical signal, the atria contracts. The signal is then passed through the atrioventricular (AV) node. After checking the signal, the AV node sends it through ventricular muscle fibers, causing them to contract. The SA node sends electrical impulses at a certain rate, but your heart rate may still change depending on physical demands, stress or hormonal factors.

## ECG TRACING OF CARDIAC CYCLE

ECG tracing of a cardiac cycle is as follows:

- P wave represents the Atrial depolarization
- QRS complex represents the Ventricular depolarization
- T wave represents the ventricular repolarization

## BLOOD VESSELS

The types of blood vessels are described below:

- <u>Arteries</u> - blood vessels that carry blood away from the heart to the body, does not have valves
- <u>Veins</u> - blood vessels that carry the blood from the body back to the heart, has valves
- <u>Capillaries</u> – one cell thick blood vessels between arteries and veins that distribute oxygen-rich blood to the body
- <u>Venules</u>- the smallest veins
- <u>Arterioles</u>- the smallest arteries.

## LAYERS OF BLOOD VESSELS

Wall of an artery consists of three (3) distinct layers of tunics

- Tunica intima- Composed of simple, squamous epithelium called endothelium. Rests on a connective tissue membrane that is rich in elastic and collagenous fibers.
- Tunica media- Makes up the bulk of the arterial wall. Includes smooth muscle fibers, which encircle the tube, and a thick layer of elastic connective tissue.
- Tunica adventitia - Consists chiefly of connective tissue with irregularly arranged elastic and collagenous fibers. This layer attaches the artery to the surrounding tissues. Also contains minute vessels (vasa vasorum--vessels of vessels) that give rise to capillaries and provide blood to the more external cells of the artery wall.

Smooth muscles in the walls of arteries and arterioles are innervated by the sympathetic branches of the autonomic nervous system. The Tunica media and the Tunica adventitia is much thicker in arteries.

## LOCATIONS OF LOWER EXTREMITY VEINS

The locations of the great saphenous, popliteal, femoral, and lesser saphenous veins are described below:

- Great saphenous- runs the entire length of the lower
- extremity and is the longest vein in the body
- Popliteal- runs deep behind the knee
- Femoral- runs deep in the upper part of the leg
- Lesser saphenous- runs lateral to the ankle, up the leg and deep behind the knee

## BEST VEIN FOR VENIPUNCTURE

First choice would be the median cubital due to its large size, and it usually doesn't bruise severely. Next choice would be the cephalic vein since it does not roll as easily as other veins. A last resort vein would be the basilica vein because it rolls easily and is positioned so that the brachial artery and a major nerve are at risk for puncture if used. Ankle and foot veins should only be punctured at the discretion of a physician and should only be used when no other veins are appropriate. Poor circulation and clotting factors may affect results of tests and cause puncture wounds that may not readily heal.

## UPPER LIMB ARTERIES

The arteries of the upper limb are described below:

- Internal thoracic - Descends posteriorly to the clavicle's sternal end and enters the thorax.
- Thyrocervical trunk - A short trunk that ascends and gives off four different branches, including the transverse and ascending cervical, and suprascapular.
- Suprascapular - Travels inferolaterally, follows the clavicle in a parallel manner, then goes posteriorly to the scapula.
- Subscapular - Descends along subscapularis muscle's lateral border to the inferior angle of the scapula.
- Thoracodorsal - Accompanies the nerve of the same name to latissimus dorsi muscle
- Deep Brachial - Accompanies the radial nerve as they pass through the humeral radial groove, then it anastomoses around the elbow joint.
- Ulnar Collateral - Anastomoses around the elbow joint.

## BLOOD AND BLOOD COMPONENTS

Blood has numerous functions – gas transport, hemostasis, defense against disease – all of which are brought about by its various components:

- <u>Red blood cells</u> – oxygen transport and gas exchange
- Blood platelets and coagulation factors – coagulation and hemostasis
- <u>Vitamin K</u> – essential cofactor in normal hepatic synthesis of some clotting factors
- <u>Plasmin</u> – lyses fibrin and fibrinogen
- <u>Antithrombin III</u> – inhibits IXa, Xa, XIa, XIIa,
- <u>Complement</u> – defense against pyogenic bacteria, activation of phagocytes, clearing of immune complexes, lytic attack on cell membranes
- <u>Lymphocytes</u> – adaptive immune response – killing of specific microbes
- <u>Monocytes</u> – respond to necrotic cell material by migrating to tissues and differentiating into macrophages
- <u>Neutrophils</u> – phagocytosis of microbes
- <u>Eosinophils</u> – phagocytosis, defense against helminthic parasites, allergic reactions
- <u>Basophils</u> – allergic reactions

## INNER WALLS OF BLOOD VESSELS

**Arteries** have three walls: The <u>tunica externa</u> is a thin layer of connective tissue that attaches the artery to tissue. The <u>tunica media</u> is the thickest layer and is composed of smooth muscle fibers and a layer of connective tissue that gives the artery elasticity. The <u>tunic interna</u> (intima) is composed of connective tissue and a layer of squamous epithelium (endothelium) that provide a smooth surface. The endothelium secretes prostacyclin, which prevents platelets from adhering to the artery walls, and other biochemicals that dilate or constrict the vessels. **Veins** also have three layers, but the middle layer is much thinner so the walls are less muscular and less elastic, and the inner diameter is greater. Some veins, especially those in the arms and legs, contain valves (flaplike) to help prevent backflow. Veins also can serve as blood reservoirs during times of blood loss, constricting to move more blood to the heart. **Capillaries**, extensions of the endothelium, are composed of a thin permeable layer of squamous epithelium through which substances in the blood are exchanged for those in tissue.

## WHOLE BLOOD, PLASMA, AND SERUM

**Whole blood** is blood as it is withdrawn from the body and contains plasma, which includes clotting factors; erythrocytes (red blood cells); leukocytes (white blood cells), which include monocytes, lymphocytes, neutrophils, basophils, and eosinophils; and thrombocytes (platelets). Whole blood is rarely used for testing or administration but is separated into components. **Plasma** is the liquid portion of the blood that is free of cells because the erythrocytes, leukocytes, and thrombocytes have been removed, but it still contains clotting factors, such as fibrinogen, because it has been treated with an anticoagulant, such as sodium citrate. **Serum**, on the other hand, is the liquid portion of blood that is also cell free but has been allowed to clot and then is spun to separate and remove the clot so that it is also free of clotting factors. Serum is more often used for testing than plasma because serum contains more antigens and can be used for a wider variety of tests. Additionally, anticoagulants found in plasma may interfere with some tests.

## RED BLOOD CELLS, WHITE BLOOD CELLS, AND PLATELETS

**Blood cells** are produced in the bone marrow. Blood is a viscous dark red fluid comprised of cells, gases, and plasma (55%). Blood components include:

- Erythrocytes (red blood cells): Red blood cells carry hemoglobin, which transports oxygen. If red blood cell count is low (such as from blood loss) or oxygen carrying capacity is impaired (such as with anemia), the patient may experience hypoxemia (low oxygen). The life cycle is normally 120 days.
- Leukocytes (white blood cells): WBCs defend the body against invading organisms (viruses, bacteria, fungi, and parasites) and in the bloodstream and tissues respond to allergies. WBCs include lymphocytes (B, T, natural killer cells, and null cells), monocytes, eosinophils, basophils and neutrophils.
- Thrombocytes (platelets): Platelets release clotting factors and have an active role in forming blood clots
- Plasma (55% of blood): Plasma carries water, proteins, electrolytes, lipids (fats), blood cells, and glucose as well as clotting factors.
- The primary blood types are A, B, AB, and O. Blood is either Rh- or RH+, and patients must receive transfusions of blood that are type and Rh compatible.

## OXYGENATION AND OXIDATION OF HEMOGLOBIN

Oxygenation is the loose, reversible binding of Hb with $O_2$ molecules forming oxyHb. Hb oxygenation is the principle method of $O_2$ uptake from the lungs into the RBCs for transport to the tissues. Each Hb molecule has the capacity to bind four $O_2$ molecules since there are four heme molecules in each Hb. $O_2$ binds loosely with the co-ordination bonds of the iron atom in the heme and not the two positive bonds of the iron. Iron is not oxidized and oxygen can be carried to the tissues in the molecular form rather than the ionic form. Oxidation of Hb involves the conversion of the functional ferrous ($Fe^{2+}$) heme iron to the non-functional ferric ($Fe^{3+}$) form. This is called methemoglobin. This oxidized form of Hb can't bind or transport oxygen. Oxidation of Hb may occur due to exposure to toxic chemicals such as nitrites, aniline dyes and oxidative drugs.

## IMMUNOGLOBULIN

The types of immunoglobulin and their functions are explained below:

- IgA– can be located in secretions and prevents viral and bacterial
- attachment to membranes.
- IgD- can be located on B cells
- IgE-main mediator of mast cells with allergen exposure.
- IgG- primarily found in secondary responses. Does cross placenta
- and destroys viruses/bacteria.
- IgM- primarily found in first response. Located on B cells

## PLASMA K+ AND ARTERIAL pH

Cells exchange K+ and H+ with plasma. In metabolic acidosis, plasma K+ concentration increases, even though body potassium may become depleted. In metabolic alkalosis, plasma K+ concentration may decrease. But although cells gain K+ initially, chronic alkalosis may result in loss of body potassium because of increased K+ excretion by renal principal cells due to increased Na+ delivery to this segment encouraging exchange of Na+ for cell K+ with K+ staying in the lumen to maintain electroneutrality. Chronic K+ depletion can result in alkalosis where decreased K+ secretion by depleted principal cells results in a greater portion of the Na+ delivered to the distal

60

tubule being reabsorbed in exchange for secreted H+ ions. The corresponding transfer of cell $HCO_3^-$ to the plasma may explain the paradoxical association of an acid urine with an alkaline plasma.

## BLOOD MOVEMENT IN THE CIRCULATORY SYSTEM

The blood flowing through the arterial system is pushed by the pressure built up by the contractions of the heart. The blood flowing through the veins relies on skeletal muscle movement to keep the valves located in the veins opening and closing to keep blood moving towards the heart and not backwards through the system.

## SKELETAL SYSTEM

### FUNCTIONS

There are about 206 bones in the human body, they function to protect and preserve the shape of soft tissues. The skeleton provides a framework for the muscles, it controls and directs internal pressure and provides stability anchoring points for other soft tissues. There are a wide variety of bones/bony tissues adapted for specific functions to aid locomotion and support; bones are moved by the skeletal muscles. In addition, the skeletal system stores and produces blood cells in the bone marrow.

> **Review Video: Skeletal System**
> Visit mometrix.com/academy and enter code: 256447

### STRUCTURES

There are two types of bone tissue: compact and spongy. The names imply that the two types of differ in density, or how tightly the tissue is packed together. There are three types of cells that contribute to bone homeostasis. Osteoblasts are bone-forming cell, osteoclasts resorb or break down bone, and osteocytes are mature bone cells. Equilibrium between osteoblasts and osteoclasts maintains bone tissue.

## BONE

### COMPACT

Compact bone is characterized by its structural components: harversian systems or closely packed osteons. Each osteon has a haversian (osteonic) central canal, which is surrounded by a matrix of lamella in concentric ring. The osteocytes (bone cells) are sandwiched between matrix rings in spaces called lacunae. Radiating out from the lacunae are small channels, called canaliculi, which connect the lacunae to the harversian canal, forming passageways through the hard matrix for transport. The harversian systems in compact bone form the appearance of a solid mass because they are so tightly packed. The harversian canals contain blood vessels running parallel to the bone's long axis. Interconnections between these blood vessels and perforating canals link vessels to those on the bone's outer surface.

### SPONGY

Compared to compact bone, spongy (cancellous) bone is lighter, airier, and less dense. Cancellous bone consists of trabeculae, which are plates and bars of bone, located adjacent to small, irregular red bone marrow-containing cavities. To receive their blood supply, the canaliculi connect with the cavities adjacent to them, rather than the central harversian canal. Although easily mistaken as a having a haphazard appearance, the trabeculae are actually arranged in a particular organization (like braces on a building) that maximizes the bone's strength. Spongy bones' trabeculae follow their bone's lines of stress and if the direction of stress changes or alters over time, the trabeculae can realign accordingly.

### OSTEOCYTES, OSTEOBLASTS, AND OSTEOCLASTS

The cells comprising bone tissue are called osteocytes, osteoblasts, and osteoclasts:

- The <u>Osteocytes</u> are found individually in spaces called lacunae within the calcified matrix of bone. They communicate with each other through small canals in the bone called canaliculi. The osteocytes in both compact and cancellous bone have a similar structure and function.
- The bone matrix is mostly formed by cells called <u>osteoblasts</u> which then sit in the matrix, transforming into osteocytes. Osteoblasts arise from mesenchymal or other undifferentiated cells. The cells are cuboidal and line the trabeculae forming in immature or developing cancellous bone.
- <u>Osteoclast</u> cells are involved in bone development and remodeling. They remove the existing mineralized bone matrix, releasing the organic and inorganic components.

## MUSCULAR SYSTEM

Muscle fibers - the specialized cells of the muscular system are contractile. Muscles are responsible for movement, whether they are attached to bones, internal organs, or blood vessels. Muscle contraction is the cause of nearly all movement in the body.

> **Review Video: Muscular System**
> Visit mometrix.com/academy and enter code: 967216

### FUNCTIONAL CHARACTERISTICS OF SKELETAL MUSCLE

The cell membrane of a muscle cell is called the sarcolemma, and it is specially structure to conduct and receive electrical impulses. The cell's sarcoplasm contains many contractile myofibrils, which relegates the nuclei and other organelles to the cell's edges. Myofibrils, contractile units within skeletal muscle cell, consist of protein myofilaments in a regular array. With respect the direction of the muscle fiber, each myofilament runs longitudinally. There are two types of myofilaments: thin filaments and thick ones. Both bands are composed of multiple molecules of a protein - actin in the thin filaments and myosin in the thick filaments. The thin actin filaments are attached to an elastic protein called titan at a Z-line or Z-disk. The titin extends into the myofibril, serving to anchor the position of the other bands. From one Z-line to the next defines a unit called a sarcomere.

### TYPES OF MUSCLE

There are three types of muscle cells in the human muscular system: skeletal, cardiac, and smooth.

- Skeletal muscles are attached to bones, enabling movement; They are under voluntary control.
- Cardiac muscle, the sole muscle type that consists of branching fibers, is striated and forms the heart.
- Smooth muscle provides movement (such as peristalsis and dilation) to the internal organs and lining of blood vessels. It is under involuntary control.

Control of movement of most muscles occurs via the nervous system, but some muscles (such as the heart) are autonomous. The human body has roughly 70,000 muscles.

## REPRODUCTIVE SYSTEM
### FUNCTIONS

The reproductive system of the human body is responsible solely for the production and utilization of reproductive cells, or gametes. The reproductive organs include reproductive organs, the reproductive tract, the perineal structures (external genitalia), and accessory glands and organs responsible for secreting fluids into the reproductive tract.

## MALE REPRODUCTIVE SYSTEM

The functions of the male reproductive system are to produce, maintain, and transfer **sperm** and **semen** into the female reproductive tract and to produce and secrete **male hormones**.

The external structure includes the penis, scrotum, and testes. The **penis**, which contains the **urethra**, can fill with blood and become erect, enabling the deposition of semen and sperm into the female reproductive tract during sexual intercourse. The **scrotum** is a sack of skin and smooth muscle that houses the testes and keeps the testes outside the body wall at a cooler, proper temperature for **spermatogenesis**. The **testes**, or testicles, are the male gonads, which produce sperm and testosterone.

The internal structure includes the epididymis, vas deferens, ejaculatory ducts, urethra, seminal vesicles, prostate gland, and bulbourethral glands. The **epididymis** stores the sperm as it matures. Mature sperm moves from the epididymis through the **vas deferens** to the **ejaculatory duct**. The **seminal vesicles** secrete alkaline fluids with proteins and mucus into the ejaculatory duct also. The **prostate gland** secretes a milky white fluid with proteins and enzymes as part of the semen. The **bulbourethral**, or Cowper's, glands secrete a fluid into the urethra to neutralize the acidity in the urethra, which would damage sperm.

Additionally, the hormones associated with the male reproductive system include **follicle-stimulating hormone (FSH)**, which stimulates spermatogenesis; **luteinizing hormone (LH)**, which stimulates testosterone production; and **testosterone**, which is responsible for the male sex characteristics. FSH and LH are gonadotropins, which stimulate the gonads (male testes and female ovaries). FSH and LH are gonadotropins, which stimulate the gonads (male testes and female ovaries).

## FEMALE REPRODUCTIVE SYSTEM

The functions of the female reproductive system are to produce **ova** (oocytes or egg cells), transfer the ova to the **fallopian tubes** for fertilization, receive the sperm from the male, and provide a protective, nourishing environment for the developing **embryo**.

The external portion of the female reproductive system includes the labia majora, labia minora, Bartholin's glands, and clitoris. The **labia majora** and the **labia minora** enclose and protect the vagina. The **Bartholin's glands** secrete a lubricating fluid. The **clitoris** contains erectile tissue and nerve endings for sensual pleasure.

The internal portion of the female reproductive system includes the ovaries, fallopian tubes, uterus, and vagina. The **ovaries**, which are the female gonads, produce the ova and secrete **estrogen** and **progesterone**. The **fallopian tubes** carry the mature egg toward the uterus. Fertilization typically occurs in the fallopian tubes. If fertilized, the egg travels to the **uterus**, where it implants in the uterine wall. The uterus protects and nourishes the developing embryo until birth. The **vagina** is a muscular tube that extends from the **cervix** of the uterus to the outside of the body. The vagina receives the semen and sperm during sexual intercourse and provides a birth canal when needed.

## URINARY SYSTEM

The urinary system's main function is to maintain the set volume and composition of fluids of the body within the bounds of their normal limits. Because a crucial role of this system is the elimination of accumulated waste products from the body that result from cellular metabolism, it is also called the excretory system. This system maintains fluid volume at appropriate levels by regulating the water volume excreted in the urine. The urinary system also regulates the concentrations of different electrolytes circulating in body fluids and maintains the blood's pH within its normal range. It also controls the production of red blood cell by secreting the hormone erythropoietin and secretes renin to help maintain normal blood pressure.

## STRUCTURES

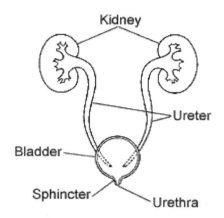

## DIGESTIVE SYSTEM

The digestive system consists of the digestive tract (that the ingested food passes through) and its the accessory organs, which assist in the chemical breakdown of food. The function of the digestive system is to process ingested food and beverages into smaller molecules that can be more readily absorbed and utilized by the body's cells. Food is broken down into increasingly smaller molecules until they can be until absorbed on a cellular level and the remaining waste eliminated. The digestive tract, termed the gastrointestinal (GI) tract or alimentary canal, is a long continuous tube extending from the mouth down to the anus. After the mouth, it passes through the pharynx and esophagus to the stomach, and then reaches the small and then large intestine. The mouth contains the accessory structures of the tongue and teeth, which help with the mechanical breaking up of food. The major accessory organs with a chemical role in digesting food include the salivary glands in the mouth, and the liver, gallbladder, and pancreas in the abdomen. These organs function to secrete fluids that help digest the food particles present in the digestive tract.

## FUNCTIONS

The following are the six main functions of the digestive system:

- <u>Ingestion</u> - The initial event in digestion is ingestion or taking in food through the mouth.
- <u>Mechanical Digestion</u> - The ingested food is in pieces that are too large for the body to use, so they must be broken down into smaller particles, increasing surface area, which various enzymes can act upon. This is the process of mechanical digestion. It begins in the mouth with mastication.

- <u>Chemical Digestion</u> - Via hydrolysis, the process of adding water and digestive enzymes to break down larger food molecules, chemical digestion transforms the complex and large molecules of carbohydrates, proteins, and fats into more readily absorbable molecules that can be used by the cells. Digestive enzymes increase the rate of hydrolysis, which is otherwise quite slow.
- <u>Movement</u> - After food is ingested and masticated, the chewed and moistened particles exit the mouth and pass through the pharynx and down the esophagus. This movement is initiated by deglutition or swallowing. In the stomach, smooth muscle contractions cause the contents to further mix together. These contractions are repetitive and occur in isolated segments of the digestive tract in succession, mixing the food with enzymes and other secretions. The rhythmic contractions that move the food particles through the alimentary canal is called peristalsis.
- <u>Absorption</u> - In the absorption process, the smaller molecules that result from the digestion process pass through the membranes of the cells lining in the walls of small intestine into the capillaries of blood or lymph vessels.
- <u>Elimination</u> - The food particles that cannot be further digested or absorbed must be eliminated. The body removes indigestible wastes in the form of feces through the anus, in the process called defecation or elimination.

## ENDOCRINE SYSTEM

The endocrine system uses chemical messengers called hormones to impact metabolic activities, growth, and development. Endocrine system actions regulate the body on a slower time table than the nervous system - more on the order of minutes, hours, days, or weeks, but both systems help maintain homeostasis. The human body has two primary categories of glands:

- <u>Exocrine Glands</u> - Include mammary, sweat, sebaceous, and digestive enzyme-secreting glands, which all contain ducts that secrete their product out to a surface.
- <u>Endocrine Glands</u> - These glands lack ducts to carry their products out to a surface; thus, they are termed ductless glands. The word "endocrine" derives from the Greek words "endo," for within, and "krine," meaning to secrete or separate.

Endocrine gland secretions are called hormones and they are released directly into the blood and then travel throughout the body. Their influence is only exerted on the cells with receptor sites for that particular hormone.

> **Review Video: <u>Endocrine System</u>**
> Visit mometrix.com/academy and enter code: 678939

## GLAND LOCATIONS

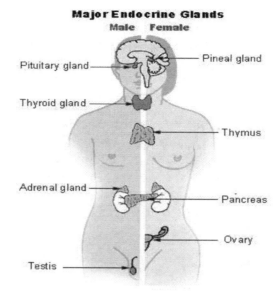

**Major Endocrine Glands**

Male   Female

Pituitary gland — Pineal gland

Thyroid gland —

Thymus

Adrenal gland —

Pancreas

Ovary

Testis —

## ALDOSTERONE LEVELS

Aldosterone is an adrenal hormone. It has a role in the regulation of water and sodium in the kidneys. A patient must be in the upright position for at least 30 minutes prior to the collection of the specimen. Also, the test is usually performed in the chemistry department.

## GROWTH HORMONE

Growth Hormone (GH), or somatotropin, is regulated by releasing and inhibiting hormones: GHRH and GHIH (called somatostatin). GH causes musculoskeletal and tissue growth and development. It stimulates the use of amino acids for protein synthesis and lipolysis to yield fatty acids to catabolize. Sometimes, it is used to stimulate muscle growth and repair and catabolize fat. GH and somatomedins (insulin-like growth factor 1) cause a negative feedback loop. These mediators are produced by the liver, muscle cells, and other tissue. Strenuous exercise and other energy-demanding activities cause a positive feedback loop. Hypersecretion of GH in childhood causes gigantism and other forms of excessive growth. Hypersecretion in adulthood causes acromegaly, which is a condition where the bones grow excessively.

## NERVOUS SYSTEM
### FUNCTIONS

The nervous system is the primary controlling, communicating, and regulatory body system. It is integral in all mental activities such as thought, memory, and learning. The nervous and endocrine systems work together to regulate and maintain homeostasis. The nervous system uses receptors to help the body respond and make sense if its internal and external environment. The three primary functions of the nervous system are motor, sensory, and integrative.

## CNS

The central nervous system (CNS) consists of the brain and spinal cord. Due to their vital importance, the brain and spinal cord and encased in bones for protection and located in the dorsal body cavity. The cranial vault houses the brain and the vertebral column's vertebral canal houses the spinal cord. Despite the fact that the brain and spinal cord are considered two separate organs, at the foramen magnum, they are continuous.

## PNS

The peripheral nervous system (PNS) consists of the nerves and ganglia. Nerves are formed from bundles of nerve fibers, similar to how muscles are formed from bundles of muscle fibers. Cranial and spinal nerves extend from the central nervous system to peripheral muscles, glands, and other structures. Ganglia are small knots or collections of nerve cell bodies located outside the central nervous system. The PNS is further subdivided into a sensory (afferent) division and a motor (efferent) division. The sensory or afferent division transmits impulses from peripheral receptors to the central nervous system. The motor or efferent division transmits impulses from the central nervous system out to peripheral muscles or organs to incite an action or effect. The motor or efferent division is further subdivided into the somatic and autonomic nervous systems. The somatic nervous system, which is also called the somatic efferent or somatomotor nervous system, functions to supply motor impulses to the body's skeletal muscles. Since these nerves afford conscious control of skeletal muscles, the system is sometimes called the voluntary nervous system. In contrast, the autonomic nervous system, which is also referred to as the visceral efferent nervous system, works to supply motor impulses to smooth and cardiac muscle, and to the epithelia of glands. It is subdivided further into two divisions: sympathetic and parasympathetic. Since the autonomic nervous system regulates functions that are involuntary or automatic, it is also called the involuntary nervous system.

## ARM NERVES

The nerves of the arms are as follows:

- Musculocutaneous Nerve - Connects to all muscles in the arm's anterior section. It becomes the lateral cutaneous nerve in the interval between the biceps and brachialis, connecting to a large area of forearm skin.
- Radial Nerve - Connects to all muscles in the arm's posterior section. With the deep brachial artery, the radial nerve descends inferolaterally around the humerus in the radial groove, further dividing into the deep and superficial branches:
- Deep Branch, for the muscles
- Superficial Branch, for the skin, but also connects to the dorsum of the hand and digits
- Median Nerve - Doesn't branch in the arm. It starts on the lateral side of the brachial artery, crossing it near the middle of the arm. It connects to most forearm flexor muscles.
- Ulnar Nerve - Doesn't branch in the arm. It runs anterior to the triceps on the medial side of the brachial artery, posterior to the medial epicondyle, and medial to the olecranon, entering the forearm.

## INTEGUMENTARY SYSTEM

The skin, the body's largest organ, is part of the integumentary system, which also is comprised of skin extensions like fingernails and hair. The skin has the vital role of protecting and cushioning the delicate organs of the body, and providing a physical barrier to keep out foreign materials out of the body and prevent it from drying out. It also helps maintain body temperature.

> **Review Video: Integumentary System**
> Visit mometrix.com/academy and enter code: 655980

## MAJOR STRUCTURES IN SKIN

Major structures found in skin:

- <u>Pore</u> -- A tiny opening in the skin that serves as an outlet for sweat
- <u>Sweat gland</u> -- Any of the glands in the skin that secrete perspiration usually located in the dermis
- <u>Nerve ending</u> -- The terminal structure of an axon that does not end at a synapse
- <u>Erector pili</u> -- Tiny smooth muscle fibers attached to each hair follicle, which contract to make the hairs stand on end
- <u>Hair follicle</u> -- A hair follicle is part of the skin that grows hair by packing old cells together. Inside the follicle the sebaceous gland is found. At the end of the hair, tiny blood vessels form the root, around the root there is a white structure called a bulb, which is visible on plucked healthy hairs.
- <u>Sebaceous gland</u> -- A gland in the skin that opens into a hair follicle and secretes an oily substance called sebum

## EPIDERMIS LAYER

As the name suggests, the epidermis, is the outermost skin layer. It has four distinct layers of epithelial tissue. The epidermis' outermost layer is the stratum corneum, which is approximately 20-30 cell layers thick. These cells are dead and completely keratinized, which forms the waterproof quality of the skin. The stratum granulosum and then the stratum lucidum are the next two layers and they are both considered to be an intermediate keratinization stage because the cells are not fully keratinized while in these layers, yet as they are pushed toward the surface when the skin grows, they become increasingly keratinized. The stratum germinativum is the deepest epidermal layer. Its cells are mitotically active, meaning they are alive and they reproduce. In this layer, the growth of skin occurs.

## DERMIS AND SUBCUTANEOUS LAYERS

- <u>Dermis</u> -- The dermis is the second layer of skin, directly beneath the epidermis. Unlike the epidermis, the dermis has its own blood supply. Sweat glands are present to collect water and various wastes from the bloodstream, and excrete them through pores in the epidermis. The dermis is also the site of hair roots, and it is here where the growth of hair takes place. By the time hair reaches the environment outside of the skin, it has died. The dermis also contains dense connective tissue, made of collagen fibers, which gives the skin much of its elasticity and strength.
- <u>Subcutaneous Layer</u> -- Beneath the dermis lays the final layer of skin, the subcutaneous layer. The most notable structures here are the large groupings of adipose tissue. The main function of the subcutaneous layer is therefore to provide a cushion for the delicate organs lying beneath the skin. It also functions to insulate the body to maintain body temperature.

## VASCULAR SYSTEM FUNCTIONS

The main functions of the vascular system include:

- Transport of cellular and chemical materials
  - Gases transported - Oxygen shuttled to the cells from the lungs and carbon dioxide (a waste product) is transported to the lungs from the cells.
  - Nutrients to cells - In addition to oxygen, other nutrients, like glucose, are transported via the circulatory system. Glucose is shuttled to the liver immediately after digestion. Glucose is used to make ATP (cellular energy) and the liver works to maintain a stable blood glucose level.
  - Cellular waste - Waste products from digestion, such as ammonia (produced from protein digestion) is transported to the liver so that it can be converted to a less toxic substance, urea, which then moves on to the kidneys, and eventually excreted in the urine.
  - Hormone transport - The vascular system transports numerous hormones that function to maintain constant internal conditions.
- Contains infection-fighting cells
- Helps stabilize body fluid pH and ionic concentration.
- Transports heat to help maintain body temperature.

## CYTOMEGALOVIRUS

Abbreviated as CMV, Cytomegalovirus is a herpes virus which can result in a life threatening situation if an infant contracts it before it is born. It can cause pneumonia or in some children result in developmental delays. CMV is tested for by an immunology test performed on serum.

## RAST

RAST is an abbreviation for the radioallergosorbent test. This test is used in the detection of allergies for example a peanut allergy.

## TUMOR MARKER

A tumor marker is a substance sometimes found in the blood, other body fluids, or tissues. A high level of tumor marker may indicate that a certain type of cancer is in the body. Examples of tumor markers include CA 125 (ovarian cancer), CA 15-3 (breast cancer), CEA (ovarian, lung, breast, pancreas, and gastrointestinal tract cancers), and PSA (prostate cancer). Tumor makers are sometimes called biomarker.

## LACTIC ACID

Lactic acid is produced by glucose-burning cells when these cells have an inadequate supply of oxygen. Lactic acid is produced in excess as a result of an oxygen deficient state called hypoxia. Examples of hypoxia are shock, hypovolemia and left ventricle failure. Excess amounts can also be caused by diabetes mellitus and toxicity. Lactic acidosis is the state where there is too much lactic acid in the blood. *Ketoacidosis ?*

## TERMS

**Pulse**: Blood vessel expansion and contraction caused by the blood pumped through them; calculated as the number of expansions occurring per minute.

**Blood Pressure**: The force exerted in the arteries by blood as it circulates. It is divided into systolic (when the heart contracts) and diastolic (when the heart is filling) pressures

**Extrasystole**: A momentary cardiac arrhythmia manifesting as premature systole, which is also called an extra heartbeat.

**Fibrillation**: Inefficient and rapid heart contraction caused by disruptions to the nerve impulses.

**Arrhythmia**: Heart contraction rate abnormalities, which may manifest as a rate that is too slow (bradycardia) or too fast (tachycardia).

**Murmur**: The noise heard between normal heart sounds, due to the flow of blood through a heart valve.

**Heart Rate**: The number of contractions of the heart in one minute. It is measured in beats per minute (bpm). When resting, the adult human heart beats at about 70 bpm (males) and 75 bpm (females), but this rate varies between people.

**Cardiac output**: The volume of blood being pumped by the heart in a minute. It is equal to the heart rate multiplied by the stroke volume.

**Stroke Volume**: The amount of blood ejected by the ventricle of the heart with each beat, usually expressed in milliliters (ml).

**Lumen**: the hollow area within a blood vessel

**Valves**: tissue flaps inside a vein or the heart that prevent backward flow of blood. Valves open as blood moves through them and close under the weight of blood collecting in the vein due to decreased pressure and gravity.

**Frontal (Coronal) Plane**: a plane parallel to the long axis of the body and perpendicular to the sagittal plane that separates the body into front and back portions.

**Sagittal Plane**: a plane that divides the body into right and left halves

**Transverse (Horizontal) Plane**: a plane that divides the body into upper and lower sections

# Medical Terminology

## ORIGIN OF MEDICAL TERMINOLOGY

Most medical terms derive from Greek or Latin, but there are a few English, French and German terms. If you break the Greek or Latin word into its root, prefix and suffix, then you can understand unfamiliar terminology. To avoid awkward pronunciation when there is no vowel between the root word and suffix, add an "o" to the combining form. For instance, add the suffix "metry" (meaning the measure of) to the root word for eye, "opt," to make the word "optometry". Examples of English terminology include: Epstein-Barr virus, HIV-positive, 100-ml sample, oxygen-dependent, or self-image. English words use a dash instead of a joining vowel. An example of French terminology is *grand mal* (the big sickness) for epileptic seizures. An example of German terminology is *mittelschmerz* (middle pain) for the discomfort of ovulation. French and German do not have convenient combining forms, so you must memorize them.

## PREFIX, ROOT, AND SUFFIX

Medical terms have three parts:

- Root containing the basic meaning
- Prefix before the root that modifies the meaning
- Suffix after the root that modifies the meaning

Examples:

- Menorrhagia is excessive bleeding during menstruation and at irregular intervals. The prefix is meno, meaning menstruation. The root is metro, meaning uterus. The suffix is rrhagia, meaning a flow that bursts forth.
- Rhinoplasty is a "nose job". The root is rhino, meaning nose. The suffix is plasty, meaning reconstructive surgery.
- Antecubitum is the bend of your arm where the nurse draws blood. The root is cubitum, meaning elbow. The prefix is ante, meaning forward or before.
- Whenever you see an unfamiliar term, break it into its root, prefix, and suffix to understand its meaning.

71

# Prefixes

| Prefix | Meaning | Example |
|--------|---------|---------|
| Ab | from, not here, off the norm | Abnormal |
| Ad | to, in the direction of | Adduct |
| Ante | prior to, in front of, previously | Antecedent |
| Anti | hostile to, against, contradictory | Antisocial |
| Be | make, aligned with, greatly | Benign |
| Bi | two, occurring twice | Bicycle |
| De | away, versus, reduce | Deduct |
| Dia | transverse, across | Diameter |
| Dis | contradictory, disparate, away | Disjointed |
| En | create, put in or on, surround | Engulf |
| Syn | by means of, together, same | Synthesis |
| Trans | across, far away, go through | Transvaginal |
| Ultra | extreme, beyond in space | Ultrasound |
| Un | opposing, antithetical, not | Uncooperative |

The following is a list of common medical terminology *prefixes*:

| Prefix | Meaning | Prefix | Meaning |
|--------|---------|--------|---------|
| A | without | Neo | new |
| An | without | Nulli | none |
| Ante | before | Pan | total |
| Bi | two | Para | beyond |
| Bin | two | Per | through |
| Brady | slow | Peri | surrounding |
| Dia | through | Poly | many |
| Dys | difficult | Post | after |
| Endo | within | Pre | before |
| Epi | over | Pro | before |
| Eu | normal | Sub | below |
| Ex | outward | Supra | superior |
| Exo | outward | Sym | join |
| Hemi | half | Syn | join |
| Hyper | excessive | Tachy | rapid |
| Hypo | deficient | Tetra | four |
| Inter | between | Trans | through |
| Intra | within | Uni | one |
| Meta | change | | |
| Micro | minute, tiny | | |
| Multi | numerous | | |

## Suffixes

| Suffix | Meaning | Example |
|---|---|---|
| -fication/-ation | manner or process | classification |
| -gram | written down or illustrated | cardiogram |
| -graph | a machine or instrument that records data | cardiograph |
| -graphy | the process of recording of data | cardiography |
| -ics | science or skill of | synthetics |
| -itis | red, inflamed, swollen | bursitis |
| -meter | means of measure | thermometer |
| -metry | action of measuring | telemetry |
| -ology/-ogy | the study of | biology |
| -phore | bearer or maker | semaphore |
| -phobia | intense, irrational fear | arachnophobia |
| -scope | instrument used for visualizing data | microscope |
| -scopy | visualize or examine | bronchoscopy |

The following is a list of common medical terminology *suffixes*:

| Suffix | Meaning | Suffix | Meaning |
|---|---|---|---|
| -ac | pertaining to | -gram | record |
| -ad | toward | -graph | recording device |
| -al | pertaining to | -graphy | process of recording |
| -algia | pain | -ia | disease condition |
| -apheresis | removal | -ial | pertaining to |
| -ar | pertaining to | -iasis | condition |
| -ary | pertaining to | -iatrist | physician |
| -asthenia | weakness | -iatry | specialty |
| -atresia | occlusion, closure | -ic | pertaining to |
| -capnia | carbon dioxide | -ician | one that |
| -cele | hernia | -ictal | attack |
| -centesis | aspirate fluid off lung | -ior | pertaining to |
| -clasia | break | -ism | condition of |
| -clasis | break | -it is | inflammation |
| -coccus | berry-like bacteria | -lysis | separating |
| -crit | separate | -malacia | softening |
| -cyte | cell | -megaly | increasing in size |
| -desis | fusion | -meter | measure |
| -drome | run | -odynia | pain |
| -eal | pertaining to | -oid | resembling |
| -ectasis | expansion | -ologist | person that practices |
| -ectomy | removal | -ology | study |
| -emia | blood dysfunction | -oma | tumor |
| -esis | condition | -opia | vision |
| -gen | agent that causes | -opsy | view of |
| -genesis | cause | -orrhagia | blood flowing profusely |
| -genic | pertaining to | | |

73

| Suffix | Meaning |
|---|---|
| -orrhaphy | repairing |
| -orrhea | flow |
| -orrhexis | break |
| -osis | condition |
| -ostomy | to make an opening |
| -otomy | cut into |
| -ous | pertaining to |
| -oxia | oxygen |
| -paresis | partial paralysis |
| -pathy | disease |
| -penia | decrease in number |
| -pepsia | digestion |
| -pexy | suspension |
| -phagia | swallowing, eating |
| -phobia | excessive fear of |
| -phonia | sound, voice |
| -physis | growth |
| -plasia | development |
| -plasm | a growth |
| -plasty | repair by surgery |
| -plegia | paralysis |
| -pnea | breathing |

| Suffix | Meaning |
|---|---|
| -poiesis | formation |
| -ptosis | sagging |
| -salpinx | fallopian tube |
| -sarcoma | malignant tumor |
| -schisis | crack |
| -sclerosis | hardening |
| -scope | visual device used for inspection |
| -scopic | visual inspection |
| -sis | condition of |
| -spasm | abnormal muscle firing |
| -stasis | standing |
| -stenosis | narrowing |
| -thorax | chest |
| -tocia | labor, birth |
| -tome | cutting device |
| -tripsy | surgical crushing |
| -trophy | develop |
| -uria | urine |

# Word Roots

The following is a list of common medical terminology *word roots*:

| Root Word | Word | Root Word | Word |
|-----------|------|-----------|------|
| abdomin/o | abdomen | cholangi/o | bile duct |
| acou/o | hearing | chol/e | gall |
| acr/o | height/extremities | chondro/o | cartilage |
| aden/o | gland | chori/o | chorion |
| adenoid/o | adenoids | chrom/o | color |
| adren/o | adrenal gland | clavic/o | clavicle |
| alveol/o | alveolus | clavicul/o | clavicle |
| amni/o | amnion | col/o | colon |
| andro/o | male | colp/o | vagina |
| angi/o | vessel | core/o | pupil |
| ankly/o | stiff | corne/o | cornea |
| anter/o | frontal | coron/o | heart |
| an/o | anus | cortic/o | cortex |
| aponeur/o | aponeurosis | cor/o | pupil |
| appendic/o | appendix | cost/o | rib |
| arche/o | beginning | crani/o | cranium |
| arteri/o | artery | cry/o | cold |
| athero/o | fatty plaque | cutane/o | skin |
| atri/o | atrium | cyan/o | blue |
| aur/I | ear | cyes/I | pregnancy |
| aur/o | ear | cyst/o | bladder |
| aut/o | self | cyt/o | cell |
| azot/o | nitrogen | dacry/o | tear |
| bacteri/o | bacteria | dermat/o | skin |
| balan/o | glans penis | derm/o | skin |
| bi/o | life | diaphragmat/o | diaphragm |
| blast/o | developing cell | dipl/o | double |
| blephar/o | eyelid | dips/o | thirst |
| bronch/I | bronchus | disk/o | disk |
| bronch/o | bronchus | dist/o | distal |
| burs/o | bursa | diverticul/o | diverticulum |
| calc/I | calcium | dors/o | back |
| cancer/o | cancer | duoden/o | duodenum |
| carcin/o | cancer | dur/o | dura |
| cardi/o | heart | ech/o | sound |
| carp/o | carpals | electr/o | electricity |
| caud/o | tail | embry/o | embryo |
| cec/o | cecum | encephal/o | brain |
| celi/o | abdomen | endocrin/o | endocrine |
| cephal/o | head | enter/o | intestine |
| cerebell/o | cerebellum | epididym/o | epididymis |
| cerebr/o | cerebrum | epiglott/o | epiglottis |
| cervic/o | cervix | episi/o | vulva |
| cheil/o | lip | epitheli/o | epithelium |

| Root Word | Word |
|---|---|
| erythr/o | red |
| esophag/o | esophagus |
| esthesi/o | sensation |
| eti/o | cause of disease |
| femor/o | femur |
| fet/I | fetus |
| fet/o | fetus |
| fibr/o | fibrous tissue |
| fibul/o | fibula |
| gangli/o | ganglion |
| ganglion/o | ganglion |
| gastr/o | stomach |
| gingiv/o | gum |
| glomerul/o | glomerulus |
| gloss/o | tongue |
| glyc/o | sugar |
| gnos/o | knowledge |
| gravid/o | pregnancy |
| gynec/o | woman |
| gyn/o | woman |
| hem/o | blood |
| hemat/o | blood |
| hepat/o | liver |
| herni/o | hernia |
| heter/o | other |
| hidr/o | sweat |
| hist/o | tissue |
| humer/o | humerus |
| hydr/o | water |
| hymen/o | hymen |
| hyster/o | uterus |
| ile/o | ileum |
| ili/o | ilium |
| infer/o | inferior |
| irid/o | iris |
| iri/o | iris |
| ischi/o | ischium |
| ischo/o | blockage |
| jejun/o | jejunum |
| kal/I | potassium |
| kary/o | nucleus |
| kerat/o | hard |
| kinesi/o | motion |
| kyph/o | hump |
| lacrim/o | tear duct |
| lact/o | milk |
| lamin/o | lamina |

| Root Word | Word |
|---|---|
| lapar/o | abdomen |
| laryng/o | larynx |
| later/o | lateral |
| lei/o | smooth |
| leuk/o | white |
| lingu/o | tongue |
| lip/o | fat |
| lith/o | stone |
| lord/o | flexed forward |
| lumb/o | lumbar |
| lymph/o | lymph |
| mamm/o | breast |
| mandibul/o | mandible |
| mast/o | breast |
| mastoid/o | mastoid |
| maxill/o | maxilla |
| meat/o | opening |
| melan/o | black |
| mening/o | meninges |
| menisc/o | meniscus |
| men/o | menstruation |
| ment/o | mind |
| metr/I | uterus |
| metr/o | uterus |
| mon/o | one |
| muc/o | mucus |
| myc/o | fungus |
| myel/o | spinal cord |
| myelon/o | bone marrow |
| myos/o | muscle |
| my/o | muscle |
| nas/o | nose |
| nat/o | birth |
| necr/o | death |
| nephr/o | kidney |
| neur/o | nerve |
| noct/I | night |
| ocul/o | eye |
| olig/o | few |
| omphal/o | navel |
| onc/o | tumor |
| onych/o | nail |
| oophor/o | ovary |
| ophthalm/o | eye |
| opt/o | vision |
| orchid/o | testicle |
| orch/o | testicle |

| Root Word | Word |
|-----------|------|
| organ/o | organ |
| or/o | mouth |
| orth/o | straight |
| oste/o | bone |
| ot/o | ear |
| ox/I | oxygen |
| pachy/o | thick |
| palat/o | palate |
| pancreat/o | pancreas |
| parathyroid/o | parathyroid gland |
| par/o | labor |
| patell/o | patella |
| path/o | disease |
| pelv/I | pelvis |
| perine/o | peritoneum |
| petr/o | stone |
| phalang/o | pharynx |
| phas/o | speech |
| phleb/o | vein |
| phot/o | light |
| phren/o | mind |
| plasm/o | plasma |
| pleur/o | pleura |
| pneumat/o | lung |
| pneum/o | lung |
| pneumon/o | lung |
| poli/o | gray matter |
| polyp/o | small growth |
| poster/o | posterior |
| prim/I | first |
| proct/o | rectum |
| prostat/o | prostate gland |
| proxim/o | proximal |
| pseud/o | fake |
| psych/o | mind |
| pub/o | pubis |
| puerper/o | childbirth |
| pulmon/o | lung |
| pupill/o | pupil |
| pyel/o | renal pelvis |
| pylor/o | pylorus |
| py/o | pus |
| quadr/I | four |
| rachi/o | spinal |
| radic/o | nerve |
| radicul/o | nerve |
| radi/o | radius |

| Root Word | Word |
|-----------|------|
| rect/o | rectum |
| ren/o | kidney |
| retin/o | retina |
| rhabd/o | striated |
| rhin/o | nose |
| rhytid/o | wrinkles |
| rhiz/o | nerve |
| salping/o | fallopian tube |
| sacr/o | sacrum |
| scapul/o | scapula |
| scler/o | sclera |
| scoli/o | curved |
| seb/o | sebum |
| sept/o | septum |
| sial/o | saliva |
| sinus/o | sinus |
| somat/o | body |
| son/o | sound |
| spermat/o | sperm |
| sphygm/o | pulse |
| spir/o | breathe |
| splen/o | spleen |
| spondyl/o | vertebra |
| staped/o | stapes |
| staphyl/o | clusters |
| stern/o | sternum |
| steth/o | chest |
| stomat/o | mouth |
| strept/o | chain-like |
| super/o | superior |
| synovi/o | synovia |
| system/o | system |
| tars/o | tarsal |
| tendin/o | tendon |
| ten/o | tendon |
| test/o | testicle |
| therm/o | heat |
| thorac/o | thorax |
| thromb/o | clot |
| thym/o | thymus |
| thyroid/o | thyroid gland |
| thyr/o | thyroid gland |
| tibi/o | tibia |
| tom/o | pressure |
| tonsill/o | tonsils |
| toxic/o | poison |
| trachel/o | trachea |

77

| Root Word | Word | Root Word | Word |
|-----------|------|-----------|------|
| trich/o | hair | vas/o | vessel |
| tympan/o | eardrum | ven/o | vein |
| uln/o | ulna | ventricul/o | ventricle |
| ungu/o | nail | ventro/o | frontal |
| ureter/o | ureter | vertebr/o | vertebra |
| urethr/o | urethra | vesic/o | bladder |
| urin/o | urine | vesicul/o | seminal vesicles |
| ur/o | urine | viscer/o | internal organs |
| uter/o | uterus | vulv/o | vulva |
| uvul/o | uvula | xanth/o | yellow |
| vagin/o | vagina | xer/o | dry |
| valv/o | valve | | |
| valvul/o | valve | | |

# Acronyms and Abbreviations

## STANDARDIZED TERMINOLOGY AND ABBREVIATIONS

Standardized terminology and abbreviations are vital for patient safety. Use abbreviations to save time and space *only when there is no potential for confusion over the meaning of your message.* Avoid Latin if there is an accepted English equivalency. Your Medical Records manager decides acceptable terminology and forbidden abbreviations. If you work in a small office and are in charge of Medical Records, use the list of safe terms from The American Society for Testing and Materials' (ASTM) and the list of dangerous abbreviations from the Institute for Safe Medication Practices (ISMP). The Joint Commission on Accreditation of Healthcare Organizations (JCAHO) also has a "Do Not Use" List for medical abbreviations and symbols that are included on the ISMP's more comprehensive list. Post them throughout your office. Use one type of units only. For example, do not use SI units (International System of Measurement) for Lab and Imperial units for Pharmacy without listing equivalencies. Adopt the U.S. Postal Service database's two-letter abbreviations for states.

Health professionals use abbreviations to save time when charting or to be discreet when speaking around a patient. Abbreviations take these forms:

- Brief form means shortening a common term or difficult to pronounce term, for example: "telephone" into "phone" and "Papanicolaou smear" into "Pap smear"
- Acronym means making word out of a phrase, for example: laser stands for light amplification by stimulated emission of radiation
- Initialism means making a word from the first letters of words in a phrase, and pronouncing the series of letters, for example, MRI for magnetic resonance imaging or HIV for human immunodeficiency virus.
- Eponym means naming a test or sign for its discoverer, for example, Coomb's test and McBurney's sign

Potentially lethal abbreviations to avoid are:

- Homonyms — Same pronunciation but different meaning, such as ileum and ilium
- Synonyms — Different words with similar meanings, such as dead and deceased

## MEDICAL ABBREVIATIONS AND ACRONYMS

| Abbreviation or Acronym | Meaning |
|---|---|
| AIDS | acquired immunodeficiency syndrome |
| A.D. | right ear, auris dextra (* on ISMP's list of error prone abbreviations) |
| A.S. | left ear, auris sinistra (* on ISMP's list of error prone abbreviations) |
| A.U. | both ears, auris utraque (* on ISMP's list of error prone abbreviations) |
| O.D. | right eye, oculus dexter (* on ISMP's list of error prone abbreviations) |
| O.S. | left eye, oculus sinister (* on ISMP's list of error prone abbreviations) |
| O.U. | both eyes, oculus uterque (* on ISMP's list of error prone abbreviations) |
| CA | cancer or carcinoma |
| CBC and diff | complete blood count and differential |
| CHF | congestive heart failure |
| TAHBSO | complete hysterectomy; total abdominal hysterectomy, bilateral salpingo-oophorectomy |
| CABG | (pronounced "cabbage") coronary artery bypass graft |

| Abbreviation or Acronym | Meaning |
|---|---|
| DNR | do not resuscitate. No codes should be called for this patient and no heroic measures should be taken to revive patient if the patient stops breathing. |
| DTR | deep tendon reflexes |
| D&C | dilatation and curettage, used to cure uterine bleeding or for early abortion |
| ECG or ECG | electrocardiogram |
| ELISA | enzyme-linked immunosorbent assay, used to test for antibodies and antigens |
| Fabere | flexion-abduction-external rotation-extension test, part of a physical to measure the patient's range of motion |
| HPI | history of present illness |
| Laser | light amplification by stimulated emission of radiation, a tool to carve tissue |
| P&A | percussion and auscultation, as in, "The lungs were clear to P&A." |
| PVH | persistent viral hepatitis |
| PND | postnasal drainage (can also mean paroxysmal nocturnal dyspnea in a sleep study) |
| simkin | simulation kinetics analysis |
| p.c. | after meals |
| a.c. | before meals |
| h.s. | bedtime |
| OD | daily [NOTE  Do not confuse with o.d., right eye.] (* on ISMP's list of error prone abbreviations) |
| ad lib | freely or whenever desired |
| p.r.n. | as needed |
| with | cum or letter c with macron |
| without | sine or letter s with a flat macron line on top |
| cm | centimeters |
| cc | cubic centimeters |
| gtt | drops |
| g | grams |
| kg | kilograms |
| q.4h. | every four hours |
| mEq | milliequivalents |

## COMMON ABBREVIATIONS

| Abbreviation | Meaning | | Abbreviation | Meaning |
|---|---|---|---|---|
| ANS | Autonomic nervous system | | C&S | Culture and sensitivity |
| | | | Ca | Calcium |
| ant | Anterior | | CBC | Completer blood count |
| ASAP | As soon as possible | | CC | Colony count |
| AV | Arteriovenous | | CEA | Carcinoma embryonic antigen |
| bid | Twice a day | | | |
| BP | Blood pressure | | Cl | Chloride |
| bpm | Beats per minute | | CNS | Central nervous system |
| BUN | Blood urea nitrogen | | CPK | Creatine phosphokinase |
| Bx | Biopsy | | CPR | Cardiopulmonary resuscitation |

| Abbreviation | Meaning |
| --- | --- |
| CSF | Cerebrospinal fluid |
| CV | Cardiovascular |
| CVP | Central venous pressure |
| D/C | Discharge |
| DW | Distilled water |
| Dx | Diagnosis |
| EBL | Estimated blood loss |
| e.m.p. | In the manner prescribed |
| ERT | Estrogen replacement therapy |
| ESR | Erythrocyte sedimentation rate |
| etiol | Etiology |
| FBS | Fasting blood sugar |
| Fe | Iron |
| FSH | Follicle-stimulating hormone |
| g | Gram |
| GERD | Gastroesophageal reflux disease |
| Grad. | Gradually |
| GTT | Glucose tolerance test |
| h | Hour |
| H or hypo. | Hypodermic |
| HD | Hemodialysis |
| H&H | Hemoglobin and hematocrit |
| Hct | Hematocrit |
| Hg | Mercury |
| Hgb | Hemoglobin |
| HIV | Human immunodeficiency virus |

| Abbreviation | Meaning |
| --- | --- |
| H&P | History and physical |
| IM | Intramuscular |
| IV | Intravenous |
| K | Potassium |
| KCL | Potassium Chloride |
| KVO | Keep Vein Open |
| lab | Laboratory |
| meds. | Medications |
| MS | Multiple Sclerosis |
| Na | Sodium |
| NB | Newborn |
| neg | Negative |
| NPO | nothing by mouth |
| O2 | Oxygen |
| OD | Overdose |
| pc | After meals |
| PCV | Packed Cell Volume |
| PM | Between noon and midnight |
| pos. | Positive |
| post-op | Postoperatively |
| PRBC | Packed Red Blood Cells |
| PSA | Prostatic specific antigen |
| PT | Prothrombin time |
| PT | Physical Therapy |
| qd | Every day |
| qod | Every other day |
| stat | Immediately |
| tid | Three times a day |

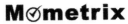

## PLURALIZING MEDICAL TERMS

Most medical laboratory terms derive from Latin and Greek. Most Latinate terms originated from the Greek. The basic rules for pluralizing medical terms are as follows:

| Rule | Example |
|------|---------|
| a changes to –ata | Stigma to stigmata<br>Condyloma to condylomata |
| -on changes to -a | Criterion to criteria<br>Phenomenon to phenomena |
| -s changes to –des | Iris to irides<br>Arthritis to arthritides |
| Feminine a ending changes to ae | Ulna to ulnae<br>Concha to conchae |
| Masculine ending us changes to i | Radius to radii<br>Musculus to musculi |
| **Rule** | **Example** |
| Neuter ending um changes to a | Bacterium to bacteria<br>Treponeum to Treponea |
| -osis changes to -oses | Diagnosis to diagnoses<br>Anastomosis to anastomoses |
| -x changes to –ces or –ges | Phalanx to phalanges<br>Varix to varices |

## MEDICAL AND SURGICAL SPECIALTIES

The suffix -ology means "the study of", and the suffix –iatrics means "medical treatment". Add the body system root to obtain the name of the specialty:

| Term | Meaning |
|------|---------|
| Anesthesiology | Study of pain relief |
| Bariatrics | Treatment of obesity |
| Cardiology | Study of the heart |
| Dermatology | Study of the skin |
| Endocrinology | Study of the hormone system |
| Gastroenterology | Study of the digestive system |
| Geriatrics | Treatment of the elderly |
| Hematology | Study of the blood |
| Neurology | Study of the nervous system |
| Obstetrics | Treatment of pregnant women |
| Pediatrics | Treatment of children |
| Psychiatry | Treatment of the mind |
| Radiology | Study of radiation (for medical imaging) |
| Rheumatology | Study of rheumatoid diseases, like arthritis |
| Toxicology | Study of poisons |
| Urology | Study of the urinary system |

## TERMS IN DOCTOR'S NOTES

| Term | Meaning |
|---|---|
| b.i.d. | twice a day |
| t.i.d | three times a day |
| q.i.d. | four times a day (* on ISMP's list of error prone abbreviations) |
| I.M. | within the muscle, intramuscular |
| I.V. | within the vein, intravenous |
| p.o. | by mouth |
| Rx | Recipe for the prescription literally means "Take thou". Also called superscription. |
| Sig | Write on the label for the patient. Also called signature. |
| STAT | immediately |
| NPO | Nihil per os (nothing by mouth), a routine precaution before surgery to prevent aspiration of vomitus. |
| Auscultation | Listening to organ sounds to make a diagnosis. Immediate auscultation uses only the ear. Mediate auscultation is with a stethoscope. |
| Diagnosis | When the doctor names or identifies the disease, judging by its signs and symptoms. |
| Palpation | Touching with the hands over the patient's skin to determine the size and consistency of underlying organs to help make the diagnosis, e.g., enlarged lymph glands, hot abdomen. |
| Percussion | Tapping the skin over an organ to determine its condition by the sound it makes. |

## REFERENCE SOURCES FOR MEDICAL TERMINOLOGY

Reliable reference sources to check correct spelling, selection and use of medical terminology are listed below:

- Abbreviations: Use safe terms and definitions from The American Society for Testing and Materials' (ASTM). Obtain a list of dangerous abbreviations to be avoided from the Institute for Safe Medication Practices.
- Style guides: Provide guidelines for format and presentation in documents. Use the *American Medical Association Manual of Style: A Guide for Authors and Editors* for an overview.
- Anatomy and physiology texts: Contain essential information regarding body structure, function of body parts, disease processes, and common health disorders. *Grey's Anatomy* is the classic.
- Specialty texts: When you need help with specialty transcriptions, try Sloan's *Medical Word Book*, Tessier's *Surgical Word Book*, and Pagana's *Laboratory and Diagnostic Tests*.
- English dictionary: Helps with spelling, definitions, and pronunciation. *Cambridge Dictionary of American English* is the standard.

# NHA Practice Test

Want to take this practice test in an online interactive format?
Check out the bonus page, which includes interactive practice questions and
much more: **https://www.mometrix.com/bonus948/nhaphleb**

**1. Transfer of an infectious agent via droplets larger than 5 μm in diameter is known as**

    a. Airborne transmission
    b. Droplet transmission
    c. Vector transmission
    d. Vehicle transmission

**2. Which of the following is an example of vector transmission?**

    a. Tuberculosis
    b. Salmonella infection
    c. Bubonic plague
    d. HIV

**3. Droplet transmission may result from**

    a. Mosquito bite
    b. Kissing
    c. Contaminated food or water
    d. Throat swab

**4. All of the following are prohibited under Centers for Disease Control (CDC) guidelines for hand hygiene EXCEPT**

    a. Hand washing using plain soap and water
    b. Artificial nails
    c. Nails longer than one quarter inch
    d. Touching faucet handles after hand washing

**5. Protective isolation may be required for all of the following patients EXCEPT**

    a. Neutropenic chemotherapy patients
    b. Burn patients
    c. Infants
    d. AIDS patients

**6. Which of the following statements regarding standard precautions for infection control is FALSE?**

    a. Use both hands to recap needles
    b. Hands should be washed before putting on and after removing gloves
    c. Standard precautions apply to all secretions except sweat
    d. Resuscitation devices may be used as an alternative to the mouth-to-mouth method

**7. Use of an N95 respirator is NOT required in the case of**
a. A child with chickenpox
b. A child with measles
c. An adult immune to measles or chickenpox
d. An adult who has never had measles or chickenpox

**8. Which of the following is NOT a violation of general laboratory safety rules?**
a. Wearing a laboratory coat when leaving the lab
b. Wearing nail polish
c. Wearing large earrings
d. Having shoulder-length hair

**9. Which of the following statements regarding HBV is FALSE?**
a. HBV vaccine also protects against HDV
b. HBV vaccine does not contain live virus
c. HBV vaccine may pose a risk of HBV transmission
d. HBV can survive up to 1 week in dried blood

**10. HCV exposure may occur through**
a. Urine
b. Sexual contact
c. Semen
d. Phlebotomy procedures

**11. To reduce the risk of transmission of a bloodborne pathogen, you should**
a. Cleanse the wound with bleach
b. Cleanse the wound with an antiseptic
c. Cleanse the wound with soap and water
d. Squeeze the wound to release fluid

**12. A specific type of fire extinguisher is used for each of the following classes of fire EXCEPT**
a. Class K
b. Class D
c. Class C
d. Class B

**13. A fire caused by the splashing of hot grease from a frying pan is classified as a**
a. Class K fire
b. Class A fire
c. Class B fire
d. Class D fire

**14. All of the following are acceptable procedures to control wound hemorrhage EXCEPT**
a. Applying direct pressure to the wound
b. Using an elastic bandage to hold the compress
c. Removing the original compress when adding additional material
d. Using cloth or gauze to apply pressure

**15. Which of the following symbols is NOT included on the Joint Commission "Do Not Use" list?**

    a.  IU

    b.  IV

    c.  U

    d.  QD

**16. Which symbol may soon be included in the Joint Commission "Do Not Use" list?**

    a.  Minus sign (-)

    b.  Equal sign (=)

    c.  Plus-or-minus sign (±)

    d.  Less than sign (<)

**17. A patient lying with his palm facing down is said to be in the**

    a.  Anatomic position

    b.  Prone position

    c.  Supine position

    d.  Reclining position

**18. Which of the following statements regarding lumbar puncture is FALSE?**

    a.  The needle enters the spinal cavity

    b.  The needle enters the space between the 3rd and 4th lumbar vertebrae

    c.  The procedure poses a risk of injury to the spinal cord

    d.  The procedure does not present a risk of spinal cord injury

**19. The hormone epinephrine**

    a.  Increases blood pressure and heart rate

    b.  Controls thyroid activity

    c.  Is associated with SAD

    d.  Decreases urine production

**20. Increased levels of which of the following are associated with heart attack?**

    a.  Albumin

    b.  PSA

    c.  CK

    d.  CEA

**21. The most frequent source of carryover contamination is**

    a.  Heparin

    b.  EDTA tubes

    c.  PTT

    d.  Coagulation tubes

**22. Which of the following is the recommended order of draw for syringes?**

    a.  The SST follows the red top

    b.  The red top follows the SST

    c.  The gray top is first

    d.  Sterile specimens are last

23. **According to the alternate order of draw for syringes,**
    a. The light-blue top is first
    b. The lavender top is first
    c. The red top and SST are last
    d. The gray top is last

24. **A sign with a picture of fall leaves may be used to indicate**
    a. Do not resuscitate order
    b. Miscarriage
    c. No blood pressures in right arm
    d. Fall precautions

25. **Which of the following statements regarding obtaining a blood specimen from a patient is FALSE?**
    a. The phlebotomist should ask the patient's permission before collecting blood
    b. The patient has the right to refuse blood draw
    c. The name of the ordering physician on the ID band should not differ
    d. Patient identity should always be verified

26. **Which of the following statements regarding patient identification is FALSE?**
    a. Outpatients may be identified by an ID card
    b. Outpatients should be asked to state their name and date of birth
    c. If a patient has been identified by the receptionist, no further verification is needed
    d. A patient's response when his or her name is called is not sufficient for identification

27. **The preferred venipuncture site is the**
    a. Cephalic vein
    b. Median cubital vein
    c. Median basilic vein
    d. Median cephalic vein

28. **All of the following statements regarding tourniquet application are true EXCEPT**
    a. The patient should be told to pump his fist
    b. A tourniquet may be applied over the patient's sleeve
    c. Two tourniquets may be used together
    d. A tourniquet should not be applied over an open sore

29. **An outpatient's blood should NOT be drawn**
    a. While reclining in a chair
    b. While lying down
    c. Unless seated in a blood-drawing chair
    d. While seated on a stool

30. **When selecting a vein for venipuncture, you should**
    a. Select a vein close to a pulse
    b. Use the basilic vein as an alternative if the median cubital vein cannot be located
    c. Palpate visible veins
    d. Use your thumb to palpate a vein

**31. If an antecubital vein cannot be located, you may**

   a. Use a vein on the underside of the wrist
   b. Perform a capillary puncture
   c. Manipulate the site until a vein can be found
   d. Use a tendon

**32. Proper technique for needle insertion includes**

   a. Pushing down on the needle
   b. Using a C hold
   c. Using an L hold
   d. Advancing the needle slowly

**33. Which of the following statements regarding blood specimens is FALSE?**

   a. Outpatient and inpatient blood specimens have the same normal values
   b. Hemoglobin and hematocrit have higher normal ranges at higher elevations
   c. Caffeine may affect cortisol levels
   d. Ingestion of butter or cheese may produce a milky specimen

**34. Blood levels of which of the following are normally lowest during the morning?**

   a. Iron
   b. Insulin
   c. Potassium
   d. Glucose

**35. Exercise increases levels of all of the following EXCEPT**

   a. Protein
   b. Cholesterol
   c. Liver enzymes
   d. Skeletal muscle enzymes

**36. All of the following affect blood specimen composition EXCEPT**

   a. Body position
   b. Temperature and humidity
   c. Fasting
   d. Stress

**37. In which of the following patients is blood collection prohibited?**

   a. Patient with a hematoma
   b. Pregnant patient
   c. Mastectomy patient
   d. Patient with a tattoo

**38. In a patient with an IV, blood should NOT be drawn**

   a. By capillary puncture
   b. Below the IV
   c. Above the IV
   d. From a different vein

**39. In obtaining a blood specimen in a patient with an IV, the phlebotomist should**

    a.  Turn off the IV

    b.  Restart the IV after venipuncture

    c.  Select a site proximal to the IV

    d.  Apply a tourniquet distal to the IV

**40. A patient begins to faint during blood collection. The most appropriate line of action would be to**

    a.  Use an ammonia inhalant to revive the patient

    b.  Continue the draw and quickly withdraw the needle

    c.  Apply pressure to the site and lower the patient's head

    d.  Allow the patient to leave after regaining consciousness

**41. All of the following may trigger hematoma EXCEPT**

    a.  Small veins

    b.  Inadequate pressure to the site

    c.  Needle penetration all the way through the vein

    d.  Petechiae

**42. To prevent hemoconcentration during venipuncture, you should**

    a.  Massage the area until a vein is located

    b.  Ask the patient to release his or her fist when blood flow begins

    c.  Ask the patient to vigorously pump his or her fist

    d.  Redirect the needle several times until a vein is located

**43. Hemolysis may result from all of the following EXCEPT**

    a.  Filling the tube until the normal amount of vacuum is exhausted

    b.  Partially filling a sodium fluoride tube

    c.  Liver disease

    d.  Pulling back the plunger too quickly

**44. Under which of the following conditions is underfilling additive tubes UNACCEPTABLE?**

    a.  When drawing blood from children

    b.  When drawing blood from anemic patients

    c.  When using a red top or SST

    d.  As a time-saving strategy

**45. Which of the following is NOT a cause of vein collapse?**

    a.  Tourniquet too close to the venipuncture site

    b.  Vacuum draw of the tube

    c.  Stoppage of blood flow on tourniquet removal

    d.  Rolling veins

**46. Capillary puncture is the preferred method for**

    a.  Dehydrated patients

    b.  Newborns

    c.  Coagulation studies

    d.  Blood cultures

**47. The recommended site for capillary puncture is the**

    a. Tip of the finger

    b. Big toe

    c. Index finger

    d. Middle finger

**48. A safe area for capillary puncture in infants is the**

    a. Medial plantar surface of the heel

    b. Posterior curvature of the heel

    c. Arch of the foot

    d. Earlobe

**49. Which of the following statements regarding warming techniques is FALSE?**

    a. Warming the site is necessary for collecting blood gas specimens

    b. Warming is required for fingersticks in patients with cold hands

    c. Warming significantly alters results of routine analyte testing

    d. Warming is recommended for heelstick procedures in infants

**50. Proper blood collection procedure includes**

    a. Wiping away the first drop of blood

    b. Applying strong repetitive pressure on the site

    c. Using a scooping motion to collect blood as it flows down the finger

    d. Removing the tube from the drop

**51. Proper procedure for capillary puncture in an infant or small child includes**

    a. Grasping only the finger to be used for puncture

    b. Grasping all of the fingers at the same time

    c. Applying a bandage after specimen collection

    d. Placing the child face down

**52. Proper procedure for TB testing includes**

    a. Applying pressure to the site

    b. Wiping the site with gauze

    c. Avoiding areas of the arm with excessive hair

    d. Applying a bandage to the site

**53. Therapeutic phlebotomy is used for all of the following EXCEPT**

    a. Polycythemia

    b. Toxicology studies

    c. Hemochromatosis

    d. Large-volume blood withdrawal

**54. Collection timing is most critical for**

    a. Phenobarbital

    b. Digoxin

    c. Ethanol

    d. Aminoglycosides

**55. Which of the following disinfectants may be used for ETOH testing?**

    a. Tincture of iodine
    b. Soap and water
    c. Isopropyl alcohol
    d. Methanol

**56. Abnormal bone function caused by a lack of vitamin D in the diet is known as**

    a. Arthritis
    b. Osteochondritis
    c. Rickets
    d. Osteomyelitis

**57. Which of the following is a form of arthritis?**

    a. Bursitis
    b. Gout
    c. Rickets
    d. Slipped disc

**58. Which of the following is used to test thyroid function?**

    a. GH
    b. GTT
    c. ADH
    d. TSH

**59. A type of diagnostic test used for cystitis is**

    a. ACTH
    b. TSH
    c. C & S
    d. FBS

**60. An individual with which type of blood can be a blood donor to individuals with any of the four blood types?**

    a. Type A
    b. Type B
    c. Type AB
    d. Type O

**61. An individual with which type of blood can receive all 4 blood types?**

    a. Type A
    b. Type B
    c. Type AB
    d. Type O

**62. The Rh factor is also known as the**

    a. A antigen
    b. B antigen
    c. AB antigen
    d. D antigen

**63. A condition marked by a decrease in the number of red blood cells is known as**

  a.  Anemia
  b.  Leukemia
  c.  Thrombocytopenia
  d.  Polycythemia

**64. The butterfly infusion set is used for all of the following types of patients EXCEPT**

  a.  Infants
  b.  Obese patients
  c.  Adults with small wrists
  d.  Elderly patients

**65. Which of the following statements regarding arterial puncture is FALSE?**

  a.  The patient should be checked for allergies before the procedure
  b.  A patient afraid of needles should be calmed down
  c.  A phlebotomist may be trained to perform the procedure
  d.  The chance of a hematoma is increased

**66. Intraoperative blood collection may be used in which type of surgery?**

  a.  Transplant
  b.  Cancer
  c.  Lower GI tract
  d.  Pediatric

**67. Which of the following statements regarding special blood collection procedures is FALSE?**

  a.  Blood pressure cannot be performed on an AV shunt
  b.  Coagulation studies cannot be drawn from a heparin lock
  c.  A heparin lock may be left in the vein for 48 hours
  d.  An implanted port should be covered with a bandage

**68. The proper pH level for arterial blood is**

  a.  5.35-5.45
  b.  7.35-7.45
  c.  3.35-3.45
  d.  2.35-2.45

**69. For blood collection with the butterfly infusion set in a child, you should use a**

  a.  23-gauge needle with a 5-mL tube
  b.  21-gauge needle with a 5-mL tube
  c.  23-gauge needle with a 2-mL tube
  d.  22-gauge needle with a 2-mL tube

**70. A normal hematocrit level for a newborn is**

  a.  42-52%
  b.  51-61%
  c.  36-48%
  d.  34-42%

71. **A patient's blood glucose level is usually elevated**

    a. After fasting
    b. After ingesting a low-carbohydrate meal
    c. After ingesting a high-carbohydrate meal
    d. Two hours after ingesting a high-carbohydrate meal

72. **The normal range for blood glucose level in a healthy adult is**

    a. 65-110 mg/dL
    b. 45-65 mg/dL
    c. 55-75 mg/dL
    d. 45-90 mg/dL

73. **All of the following are blood gas values EXCEPT**

    a. pH
    b. BUN
    c. $pCO_2$
    d. Hct

74. **The most plentiful electrolyte in serum or plasma is**

    a. Potassium
    b. Sodium
    c. Chloride
    d. Calcium

75. **Both sodium and potassium play a major role in**

    a. Osmotic pressure
    b. Muscle function
    c. Cardiac output
    d. Renal function

76. **Which of the following statements regarding HCG testing is FALSE?**

    a. Contaminants such as detergent may invalidate results
    b. Medications may produce false-negative results
    c. Positive results are available the first week after conception
    d. Ovarian tumors may increase levels

77. **Which of the following characteristics of a urine sample is indicative of a pathological condition?**

    a. White or pigmented yellow foam
    b. Dark amber color
    c. Epithelial cells
    d. Bacteria

78. **A urine sample is considered acidic at a pH of**

    a. 7
    b. Less than 7
    c. Greater than 7
    d. 3

93

**79. All of the following are indicative of a UTI EXCEPT**

    a. Leukocytes
    b. Nitrites
    c. Protein
    d. Glucose

**80. Trough levels are collected**

    a. 30 to 60 minutes after the drug is administered
    b. To screen for drug intoxication
    c. Prior to administration of the next dose
    d. For DNA testing

**81. TB is diagnosed using the**

    a. Schick test
    b. PPD test
    c. Dick test
    d. Histo test

**82. All of the following cannot be ingested prior to a fecal occult blood test EXCEPT**

    a. Vitamin C
    b. Aspirin
    c. Spinach
    d. Horseradish

**83. Which of the following is NOT normally present in the urine?**

    a. Ketones
    b. Bilirubin
    c. Albumin
    d. Bacteria

**84. Which of the following specimens must be kept at or near body temperature?**

    a. Lactic acid
    b. Ammonia
    c. Glucagon
    d. Cryoglobulin

**85. The ___ plane divides the body into top and bottom halves.**

    a. Sagittal
    b. Midsagittal
    c. Transverse
    d. Frontal

**86. The abbreviation Q2H indicates that the drug should be given**

    a. Twice a day
    b. Every hour
    c. By mouth
    d. Every 2 hours

**87. The most common type of tissue found in the body is**

   a. Connective
   b. Muscle
   c. Epithelial
   d. Nerve

**88. The total number of bones in the body is**

   a. 200
   b. 100
   c. 206
   d. 106

**89. The total number of muscles in the body is**

   a. 566
   b. 656
   c. 556
   d. 560

**90. The area between neurons over which impulses jump is known as the**

   a. Axon
   b. Dendrite
   c. Synapse
   d. Myelin sheath

**91. The gray matter of the brain is composed of**

   a. Myelin sheath
   b. Nonmyelinated axons
   c. Schwann cells
   d. Synapses

**92. The PNS is composed of**

   a. Cranial nerves
   b. Optic nerves
   c. Spinal cord
   d. CNS

**93. Hydrocephalus is characterized by**

   a. Stiff neck
   b. Nerve pain
   c. Shuffling gait
   d. Enlarged head

**94. The outermost layer of the skin is known as the**

   a. Dermis
   b. Epidermis
   c. Subcutaneous layer
   d. Hypodermal layer

**95. A condition characterized by protrusion of the stomach is known as**

a. Gastritis
b. GERD
c. Hiatal hernia
d. Peptic ulcer

**96. The ___ is a type of exocrine gland.**

a. Pancreas
b. Pituitary
c. Thyroid
d. Sweat gland

**97. Which of the following conditions is caused by dysfunction of the pituitary gland?**

a. Cushing syndrome
b. Dwarfism
c. Diabetes
d. Parkinson disease

**98. The throat is also known as the**

a. Trachea
b. Larynx
c. Pharynx
d. Epiglottis

**99. Asthma is caused by**

a. Obstruction of the airway
b. Inflammation of the bronchial tubes
c. Too rapid breathing
d. Oxygen deficiency

**100. The major portion of the heart is known as**

a. Endocardium
b. Pericardium
c. Myocardium
d. Atrium

**101. The pumping chambers of the heart are known as the**

a. Ventricles
b. Atria
c. Endocardium
d. Septum

**102. The human body has an average of ___ pints of blood.**

a. 4-5
b. 10-12
c. 8-10
d. 6-8

**103. Approximately 92% of plasma is composed of**

    a. Fibrinogen
    b. Solutes
    c. Electrolytes
    d. Water

**104. A typical diagnostic test for cardiovascular disease is**

    a. CBC
    b. Hgb
    c. AST
    d. ESR

**105. The site typically used for testing ABGs is the**

    a. Venous puncture
    b. Arterial puncture
    c. Antecubital vein
    d. Median cubital vein

**106. Which type of urine specimen collection method is used in small children?**

    a. Clean catch
    b. Midstream clean catch
    c. Suprapubic
    d. Regular void

**107. All of the following may be used to test the CSF EXCEPT**

    a. Chloride
    b. Total protein
    c. Glucose
    d. ABO

**108. This specimen is collected 2 hours after the patient has ingested a meal**

    a. FBS
    b. PP
    c. Hgb
    d. HBV

**109. All of the following can affect GTT results EXCEPT**

    a. Aspirin
    b. Birth control pills
    c. Corticosteroids
    d. Blood pressure medications

**110. Which of the following is NOT used for coagulation monitoring?**

    a. ACT
    b. Hgb
    c. PT
    d. PTT

**111. Which of the following tests may be performed together to assess clotting abnormalities?**

    a.   ACT and PT

    b.   ACT and APPT

    c.   PT and PTT

    d.   PT and PP

**112. Which of the following statements regarding the APPT test is FALSE?**

    a.   Plasma values of 24 to 34 seconds are considered normal

    b.   Whole blood values are the same as plasma values

    c.   Whole blood values between 93 and 127 seconds are considered normal

    d.   Plasma values differ from whole blood values

**113. Which of the following tests is typically ordered stat?**

    a.   $pCO_2$

    b.   HCG

    c.   FBS

    d.   Hgb

**114. Enteric isolation procedures are required for**

    a.   Patients with tuberculosis

    b.   Burn patients

    c.   Patients with intestinal infections

    d.   Patients with skin infections

**115. OSHA requires that a HEPA respirator be used for**

    a.   Enteric isolation

    b.   Burn patients

    c.   Contact isolation

    d.   AFB patients

**116. SDS is required by OSHA for**

    a.   Bloodborne pathogens

    b.   Electrical hazards

    c.   Hazardous chemicals

    d.   Radioactive hazards

**117. Which of the following is NOT part of standard safety procedure?**

    a.   Recapping contaminated needles

    b.   Replacing bed rails after specimen collection

    c.   Reporting items dropped on the floor

    d.   Reporting unusual odors

**118. All of the following are required for pathogen growth EXCEPT**

    a.   Water

    b.   Proper pH

    c.   Heat

    d.   Darkness

**119. Postexposure treatment is recommended for**

a. HCV
b. HBV
c. HIV
d. HBIG

**120. Which of the following statements regarding HIV is FALSE?**

a. HIV may be transmitted through breast milk
b. No vaccine is available for HIV
c. Postexposure treatment is recommended for occupational exposures
d. Those exposed to HIV must be retested 6 months after exposure

**121. The source of transmission of a pathogen to others is known as the**

a. Susceptible host
b. Reservoir host
c. Direct contact
d. Chain of infection

**122. PPE is NOT required when entering the room of a patient with**

a. Skin infection
b. Tuberculosis
c. Intestinal infection
d. HIV

**123. Which of the following statements regarding laboratory hazards is FALSE?**

a. Lead aprons should be worn as a precaution for radioactive hazards
b. Mixing bleach and ammonia creates a chemical hazard
c. All chemical exposures require flushing the eyes or affected parts with water
d. Electrical hazards should be removed using a broom handle

**124. Which of the following information is NOT required on specimen tube labels?**

a. Accession number
b. Physician's signature
c. Phlebotomist's initials
d. Time of test

**125. All of the following are used to send laboratory requisition forms to the lab EXCEPT**

a. Courier
b. Pneumatic tubes
c. E-mail
d. Verbal laboratory request

**126. Which of the following statements regarding health care communication is FALSE?**

a. Comfort zones are dependent on culture
b. Callers should not be put on hold
c. Sign language may be used for hearing-impaired patients
d. Sign language may be used for non–English-speaking patients

**127. Which of the following constitutes negligence?**

   a. Intent to harm
   b. Invasion of privacy
   c. Injury
   d. Abandonment

**128. An example of an intentional tort is**

   a. Abandonment
   b. Negligence
   c. Malpractice
   d. Chain of custody

**129. Pre- and post- are examples of**

   a. Abbreviations
   b. Suffixes
   c. Prefixes
   d. Root words

**130. The term caudal means**

   a. Toward the midline
   b. Toward the side
   c. Toward the head
   d. Toward the tail

**131. Which of the following is NOT required for drug or alcohol testing?**

   a. Patient consent
   b. Split sample
   c. Plastic tube
   d. Proctor

**132. Bleeding time may be decreased by**

   a. Blood pressure
   b. Aspirin
   c. Ethanol
   d. Dextran

**133. The ACT test is used to monitor**

   a. $PO_2$
   b. Heparin
   c. Ionized calcium
   d. Glucose

**134. All of the following are trace elements EXCEPT**

   a. Arsenic
   b. Zinc
   c. Iron
   d. Magnesium

## 135. Troponin is used in the diagnosis of

a. Diabetes
b. Heart attack
c. Anemia
d. Colon cancer

## 136. All of the following are skin tests EXCEPT

a. PPD
b. Histo
c. BNP
d. Cocci

## 137. In administering a TB test,

a. The antigen must be injected into a vein
b. The antigen must be injected just below the skin
c. The degree of erythema is measured to determine a reaction
d. Presence of a bleb or wheal indicates the antigen was injected improperly

## 138. A positive reaction to a TB test is indicated by

a. Induration between 5 and 9 mm in diameter
b. Induration less than 5 mm in diameter
c. Induration greater than 10 mm in diameter
d. Degree of erythema

## 139. All of the following are included in the procedure for strep testing EXCEPT

a. Latex agglutination
b. Nitrous acid extraction
c. Enzyme immunoassay
d. Specific gravity

## 140. Which of the following statements regarding arterial puncture is FALSE?

a. Arterial puncture is more difficult to perform than venipuncture
b. Arterial puncture is used to evaluate ABGs
c. Arterial puncture is used for routine blood tests
d. Arterial puncture is more painful than venipuncture

## 141. Decreased levels in the blood, as measured by one of the following, increase the respiration rate.

a. $PCO_2$
b. $PO_2$
c. $HCO_3$
d. pH

## 142. Base excess or deficit is calculated based on all of the following EXCEPT

a. $PCO_2$
b. $HCO_3$
c. Hct
d. $O_2$ saturation

### 143. Which of the following statements regarding the radial artery is FALSE?

a. The radial artery may be difficult to locate in patients with low cardiac output
b. If the radial artery is damaged, the ulnar artery may be used for arterial puncture
c. The radial artery should not be punctured in the absence of collateral circulation
d. The radial artery carries a higher risk of hematoma

### 144. The femoral artery is located in the

a. Groin
b. Scalp
c. Arm
d. Umbilical cord

### 145. In performing the Allen test,

a. The patient should hyperextend the fingers
b. Blanching of the hand indicates a positive result
c. Both the radial and ulnar arteries should be compressed at the same time
d. Only the radial artery should be compressed

### 146. In infants, which of the following sites may be used for arterial puncture?

a. Brachial artery
b. Umbilical artery
c. Femoral artery
d. Ulnar artery

### 147. The presence of a wheal indicates

a. Proper injection of a local anesthetic
b. Positive TB test
c. Positive Allen test
d. Improper injection of the TB antigen

### 148. The vasovagal response is commonly known as

a. Allergic reaction
b. Myocardial infarction
c. Fainting
d. Hematoma

### 149. Serous fluid may be obtained from all of the following EXCEPT the

a. Peritoneal cavity
b. Pleural cavity
c. Pericardial cavity
d. Spinal cavity

### 150. The C-urea breath test is used to detect

a. Lactose intolerance
b. *H pylori*
c. Trace metals
d. Blood disorders

# Answer Key and Explanations

**1. B:** Droplet transmission involves transfer of an infectious agent via droplets larger than 5 μm in diameter, whereas airborne transmission involves dispersal of infectious evaporated droplet nuclei less than 5 μm in diameter. In vector transmission, infectious agents are carried by insects, arthropods, or animals; in vehicle transmission, infectious agents are transmitted through contaminated food, water, or drugs.

**2. C:** The transmission of bubonic plague by fleas from rodents is an example of vector transmission; tuberculosis is spread via airborne transmission. Transmission of salmonella infection associated with handling contaminated food and human immunodeficiency virus (HIV) infection through blood transfusion are examples of vehicle transmission.

**3. D:** Droplet transmission may result from transfer of infectious agents by coughing, sneezing, or talking or through procedures such as throat swab collection. Vector transmission may result from mosquito or flea bites and vehicle transmission though contaminated food or water; transfer of an infectious agent through kissing or touching is known as direct contact transmission.

**4. A:** Routine hand washing using plain soap and water is required to prevent spread of infection; alcohol-based antiseptic hand cleaners may also be used. Artificial nails or nails longer than one quarter inch are prohibited. After hand washing, a clean paper towel should be used to turn off the faucet to prevent contamination.

**5. C:** Protective or reverse isolation may be required for patients highly susceptible to infection, such as burn patients, patients with AIDS, or chemotherapy patients with a low neutrophil count; protective isolation is usually not required for infants.

**6. A:** Never use both hands to recap a needle; hands should be washed both before putting on and after removing gloves. Standard precautions should be followed for all body fluids except sweat; resuscitation devices may be used as an alternative to mouth-to-mouth resuscitation.

**7. C:** An N95 respirator must be worn by all individuals susceptible to measles or chickenpox before entering the room of a patient known or suspected to have these diseases; however, adults who are immune to measles or chickenpox are not required to wear an N95 respirator or surgical mask.

**8. D:** Shoulder-length or longer hair is acceptable in the laboratory if it is tied back; wearing nail polish or large or dangling earrings is not acceptable. A laboratory coat should never be worn when leaving the lab for any reason.

**9. C:** HBV vaccine does not contain live virus and thus does not carry the risk of HBV infection; HBV vaccine also protects against hepatitis D virus (HDV) because it is only contracted concurrently with HBV. HBV can survive up to 1 week in dried blood on work surfaces or other objects.

**10. B:** Hepatitis C virus (HCV) infection may occur through exposure to blood and serum and is primarily transmitted through sexual contact and needle sharing; however, it is rarely found in urine or semen and is not associated with phlebotomy procedures.

**11. C:** Cleansing the wound with plain soap and water for at least 30 seconds is useful in reducing the risk of transmission of a bloodborne pathogen; squeezing the wound or cleansing the wound with an antiseptic, bleach, or other caustic agents is not recommended.

**12. B:** A specific class of fire extinguisher is used for each class of fire except for class D fires; these types of fires involve combustible or reactive metals such as sodium, potassium, magnesium, or lithium and should be handled by trained firefighting personnel.

**13. A:** Class K fires are often caused by high-temperature cooking oils, grease, or fats; class A fires occur with wood, paper, or clothing and class B fires with flammable liquids and vapors such as paint or gasoline. Class D fires are associated with combustible or reactive materials such as sodium or potassium.

**14. C:** When adding additional compresses to a wound, the original compress should not be removed to avoid interference with the clotting process; direct pressure should be applied to the wound using cloth or gauze. An elastic bandage can be used to hold the compress in place.

**15. B:** IV is an acceptable acronym; however, IU, or international unit, is often confused with IV and thus should not be used. U should be written out as "unit" and QD as "daily."

**16. D:** The symbols for less than ($<$) and greater than ($>$) are often confused for the letter "L" and the number 7, respectively, and thus may soon be added to the "Do Not Use" list.

**17. B:** A patient lying face down or with his palm facing down is in the prone position; a patient lying on his back with his face up is in the supine position. A patient standing erect with arms at his sides and palms facing forward is in the anatomic position.

**18. C:** Because the spinal cord ends at the first lumbar vertebra, lumbar puncture does not present a risk of spinal cord injury. The physician inserts the needle into the spinal cavity at the space between the 3rd and 4th lumbar vertebrae.

**19. A:** The hormone epinephrine increases heart rate, blood pressure, and metabolic rate; the antidiuretic hormone (ADH) decreases urine production and calcitonin lowers blood calcium levels. Melatonin helps set diurnal rhythms and is associated with seasonal affective disorder (SAD).

**20. C:** Increased levels of creatine kinase (CK) are associated with heart attack; PSA, or prostate specific antigen, level is used to test for prostate cancer. Carcinoembryonic antigen (CEA) is used in digestive system testing and albumin in urinary system testing.

**21. B:** EDTA tubes are more frequently associated with carryover contamination than any other types of additives, while heparin is associated with the least amount of interference. Coagulation tubes are the first to be used because all other additive tubes interfere with coagulation tests; partial thromboplastin time (PTT) tests are affected by tissue thromboplastin contamination.

**22. A:** In the recommended order of draw for syringes, sterile specimens are first, followed by light-blue tops; the SST follows the red top and the gray-top tube is last.

**23. C:** According to the alternate syringe order of draw, the sterile specimens remain first, while the red top and SST tubes are last.

**24. D:** A sign with a picture of falling leaves indicates that fall precautions are required for the patient. The letters DNR indicate a do not resuscitate order, and a sign depicting a delete symbol over an arm with a needlestick indicates no blood pressures in right arm.

**25. C:** Occasionally, the name of the ordering physician, room number, or bed number on the patient's ID band may differ; however, patient identity must always be verified before collecting blood. As part of informed consent, patients have the right to refuse blood draw; thus, the phlebotomist must ask the patient's permission before collecting blood.

**26. C:** The phlebotomist should always verify a patient's ID, even if he or she has been identified by the receptionist or has responded when his or her name has been called. Some outpatients may have been issued an ID card by the clinic; however, outpatients should still be asked to confirm their name and date of birth.

**27. B:** Because the median cubital vein is closer to the surface and located in an area least prone to nerve damage, it is the preferred site for venipuncture. The cephalic and median cephalic veins are the second choice; the basilic and median basilic veins are least preferred because of their proximity to the median nerve and brachial artery.

**28. A:** When applying a tourniquet, fist pumping should be discouraged, as it may make vein location more difficult or cause changes in blood components that may affect test results. A tourniquet may be applied over a patient's sleeve if the sleeve is too tight and cannot be rolled up far enough; a tourniquet should never be placed over an open sore. Because a tourniquet may have a tendency to roll or twist on the arm of an obese patient, two tourniquets may be placed on top of each other and used together.

**29. D:** Blood drawing should not be performed on an outpatient who is standing or seated on a high or backless stool because of the possibility of fainting. Outpatients should be seated on a special blood-drawing chair or on a chair with armrests; however, if the patient has a tendency to faint, he or she may be seated in a reclining chair or lying down.

**30. C:** In selecting a vein for venipuncture, even visible veins should be palpated to judge suitability for venipuncture. If the median cubital vein cannot be located, the basilic vein should not be used unless no other vein is more prominent because of the possibility of nerve injury or damage to the brachial artery. Do not use veins that overlie or are located close to a pulse to avoid the risk of puncturing an artery. The thumb should not be used because it has a pulse and may cause a vein to be mistaken for an artery.

**31. B:** If an antecubital vein cannot be found on either arm, a capillary puncture may be considered provided the test can be performed on capillary blood. Veins on the underside of the wrist should not be used to avoid nerve injury; tendons should not be used as they are difficult to penetrate and lack resilience. Manipulating the site may change blood composition, which may interfere with test results.

**32. C:** The proper technique for anchoring the vein before venipuncture is known as the L hold technique, which involves using the fingers to support the back of the patient's arm below the elbow and placing the thumb 1 to 2 inches and slightly to the side of the venipuncture site to pull the patient's skin toward the wrist; the C hold technique, or the two-finger technique, should not be used as it may result in the needle springing back into the phlebotomist's index finger if the patient pulls his or her arm back. Pushing down on the needle during insertion is painful and may increase the risk of blood leakage; advancing the needle too slowly may prolong the patient's discomfort.

**33. A:** Because outpatient specimens are not obtained during the basal state, normal values may differ slightly from those of inpatients; hemoglobin (Hgb), hematocrit (Hct), and red blood cell (RBC) counts may have higher normal ranges at higher elevations. Caffeinated beverages may affect cortisol levels; ingestion of lipids such as butter or cheese may increase blood lipid content, giving blood specimens a cloudy or milky appearance.

**34. D:** Blood glucose levels are usually lowest in the morning; however, iron, insulin, and potassium levels are usually highest in the morning.

**35. C:** Exercise may increase levels of protein, insulin, glucose, and cholesterol, as well as skeletal muscle enzyme levels, but does not affect liver enzyme levels.

**36. C:** Body position, environmental conditions such as temperature and humidity, and stress can affect blood specimen composition; fasting is useful in eliminating dietary influences on blood testing.

**37. A:** Venipuncture should never be performed through a hematoma; if there is no alternative, an area distal to the hematoma should be used. In patients with a tattoo, it is best to choose another site; however, if there is no alternative, the needle should be inserted in an area that does not contain dye. In a mastectomy patient, blood should not be drawn from the arm on the same side of the mastectomy, but can be drawn from the other arm. Pregnancy does not preclude blood collection.

**38. C:** In a patient with an IV, blood should never be drawn from a site above the IV, as the specimen may become contaminated with IV fluid, causing erroneous test results. Venipuncture can be performed at a site distal to the IV, in a different vein than the one with the IV, or by capillary puncture.

**39. D:** A phlebotomist is not qualified to start or adjust an IV; rather, he or she should ask the nurse to turn off the IV at least 2 minutes before blood collection and restart the IV after venipuncture. A site distal to the IV should always be selected for venipuncture.

**40. C:** If a patient faints during blood collection, discontinue the draw and discard the needle; pressure should be applied to the site to prevent bleeding and bruising and the patient should be asked to lower his or her head and breathe deeply to allow oxygenated blood to access the brain. Ammonia inhalants may produce side effects such as respiratory distress in asthmatic patients and should not be used. After he or she regains consciousness, the patient should remain in the room for at least 15 minutes.

**41. D:** Petechiae, or small red spots that appear on the patient's skin when the tourniquet is applied, are usually caused by capillary wall defects or platelet abnormalities and are indicative of heavy bleeding at the venipuncture site; however, they are not indicative of hematoma. Using veins that are too small or fragile for the size of the needle, applying inadequate pressure to the site, and allowing the needle to penetrate all the way through the vein may cause hematoma formation.

**42. B:** To prevent hemoconcentration during venipuncture, the phlebotomist should ask the patient to release his or her fist when blood begins to flow; fist pumping may increase blood potassium levels and should not be encouraged. Excessively massaging the site or probing or redirecting the needle multiple times may result in hemoconcentration.

**43. A:** Evacuated tube system (ETS) tubes should always be filled until the normal amount of vacuum is exhausted; partially filling a normal draw sodium fluoride tube or pulling back the plunger on a syringe too quickly may result in hemolysis. Although procedural errors are the most common cause, patient conditions such as liver disease or hemolytic anemia may result in hemolysis.

**44. D:** Underfilling additive tubes is unacceptable as a time-saving device; underfilling is acceptable when obtaining larger amounts of blood is inadvisable, such as when drawing blood from infants or children or from severely anemic patients. Short draw serum tubes such as red tops and serum separator tubes (SSTs) are acceptable provided the specimen is not hemolyzed and there is enough of the specimen for testing.

**45. C:** A collapsed vein may result from the vacuum draw of the tube or pressure from pulling on the syringe or if the tourniquet is too tight or too close to the venipuncture site. Stoppage of blood flow when the tourniquet is removed may simply indicate that the needle is not positioned properly; slightly adjusting the needle usually reestablishes blood flow. Improper needle position may result in rolling veins.

**46. B:** Capillary puncture is the preferred method for infants and young children due to their smaller blood volume and risk of injury or serious adverse events such as anemia or cardiac arrest and is typically used for newborn screening; however, it is not appropriate for dehydrated patients or those with poor circulation. Capillary puncture cannot be used for coagulation studies, blood cultures, or tests requiring large volumes of serum or plasma.

**47. D:** The middle or ring finger is the recommended site for capillary puncture; the tip of the finger should not be used due to the short distance between the skin surface and bone nor the index finger because of its increased sensitivity and more frequent use. The big toe is no longer recommended as a site for capillary collection.

**48. A:** The medial or lateral plantar surface of the heel is the preferred site for capillary puncture; the earlobe or arch or other areas of the foot should not be used for puncture. The posterior curvature of the heel should not be used, as the bone may be only 1 mm deep in this area.

**49. C:** Warming of the injection site does not significantly affect results of routinely tested analytes; warming is preferred for heelstick procedures in infants due to their high red blood cell counts and is required for collection of blood gas or capillary pH specimens. Warming may be required before fingersticks in patients with cold hands.

**50. A:** During blood collection, the first drop of blood should be wiped away, as it may be contaminated with tissue fluid or may contain alcohol residue that may hemolyze the specimen or prevent blood from forming a well-rounded drop. Using strong repetitive pressure to milk the site may result in hemolysis or tissue fluid contamination; using a scooping motion against the skin surface may cause platelet clumping or hemolysis. Removing the tube from the site may create air spaces in the specimen that interfere with test results.

**51. B:** In performing a capillary puncture in an infant or small child, grasp all of the child's fingers between your fingers and thumb; grasping only one finger may cause the finger to twist if the child tries to pulls away. Bandages should not be applied to infants or children younger than 2 years of age as they may present a choking hazard or may stick and cause the skin to tear during removal. For heelstick procedures, the infant or child should be lying face up with the foot lower than the torso.

**52. C:** When administering a tuberculosis (TB) skin test, avoid areas of the arm with scars, bruises, burns, or excessive hair because they may interfere with test results. Applying pressure to the site may force the antigen out of the site and wiping the site with gauze may cause the antigen to be absorbed. Applying a bandage to the site may result in fluid absorption or irritation and may affect test results.

**107**

**53. B:** Therapeutic phlebotomy is the withdrawal of large volumes of blood and may be used as treatment for certain conditions such as polycythemia or hemochromatosis; it is not used for toxicology, or the study of toxins or poisons.

**54. D:** Collection timing is most critical for drugs with short half-lives, such as the aminoglycosides; timing is less critical for drugs with longer half-lives such as phenobarbital or digoxin. Timing is not essential for ethanol or blood alcohol testing.

**55. B:** During blood alcohol (ethanol) [ETOH] testing, regular soap and water may be used to clean the venipuncture site if an alternative disinfectant such as povidone-iodine or aqueous benzalkonium chloride is not available; disinfectants that contain alcohol such as tincture of iodine, isopropyl alcohol, or methanol should not be used, as they may compromise test results.

**56. C:** Rickets usually occurs in children and is marked by abnormal or "soft" bones caused by a lack of vitamin D in the diet; arthritis is an inflammatory condition of the joints. Osteochondritis is an inflammation of the bone and cartilage, and osteomyelitis is inflammation of the bone or bone marrow caused by bacterial infection.

**57. B:** Gout is a form of arthritis affecting the joints of the feet caused by increased uric acid levels in the blood; bursitis is an inflammation of the bursa between the muscle attachments and bone. Rickets is a condition in children caused by lack of vitamin D marked by softening and malformation of the bones; a slipped disc is a condition in which the disc between the vertebrae of the spine ruptures or protrudes out of place.

**58. D:** The thyroid-stimulating hormone (TSH) test is used to assess thyroid function; GH stands for growth hormone, and ADH stands for antidiuretic hormone. GTT is the glucose tolerance test.

**59. C:** The urine culture and sensitivity (C & S) test is used to diagnose cystitis; ACTH is used to assess adrenocorticotropic hormone and thyroid-stimulating hormone (TSH) levels. FBS is the fasting blood sugar test.

**60. D:** Because type O blood lacks antigens, an individual with type O blood can be a donor to individuals with any of the four blood types; thus, type O blood is known as the universal donor.

**61. C:** Because type AB blood lacks antibodies in its plasma, an individual with this blood type can receive blood from all 4 blood types; thus, type AB blood is known as the universal recipient.

**62. D:** The Rh factor is also known as the D antigen.

**63. A:** Anemia is a condition indicated by a deficiency of red blood cells and hemoglobin in the blood; leukemia is a condition characterized by an increase in the number of white blood cells. Thrombocytopenia is marked by a decrease in the number of platelets and polycythemia an excessive number of red blood cells.

**64. B:** The butterfly infusion set is used for patients with small, fragile veins, such as the elderly, infants or small children, or adults with small antecubital wrists; it is not used in obese patients.

**65. C:** Only physicians or specially trained emergency room personnel are qualified to perform arterial puncture; the phlebotomist is not trained to perform this procedure. Patients should be checked for allergies and must be in a steady state; thus, a patient who is afraid of needles must be calmed down before the procedure. The risk of hematoma is increased with arterial puncture.

**66. A:** Intraoperative blood collection is used for procedures in which the estimated amount of blood loss is 20% or more of the patient's blood volume; it is typically used in patients undergoing cardiac, vascular, gynecologic, trauma, or transplant surgery. Intraoperative blood collection is not used for cancer or lower GI tract surgery or for infants or small children due to the risk of anemia or cardiac arrest.

**67. D:** An implanted port is attached to an indwelling line and should not be covered with a bandage. A heparin lock is a special type of cannula that can be left in the patient's vein for up to 48 hours; however, coagulation studies should not be drawn from a heparin lock. Arteriovenous (AV) shunts are usually created to provide access for dialysis; venipuncture or blood pressure should not be performed on an AV shunt.

**68. B:** The pH for arterial blood should be maintained at a level of 7.35 to 7.45.

**69. C:** For a pediatric patient, a 23-gauge needle with a 2-mL tube should be used for butterfly infusion; use of a 5-mL tube with a 23-gauge needle may cause vein collapse or hemolysis of the specimen.

**70. B:** The normal hematocrit (Hct) for a newborn is within the range of 51% to 61%. For a male adult, the range should be 42% to 52%, for a female adult, 36% to 48%, and for a 6-year-old child, 34% to 42%.

**71. C:** A patient's blood glucose level is normally elevated after ingestion of a high-carbohydrate meal; however, glucose levels return to normal within 2 hours after ingestion.

**72. A:** Normal blood glucose levels for a healthy adult should range from 65 to 110 mg/dL.

**73. D:** Although values for hematocrit (Hct) are measured through a chemistry panel, Hct is not a blood gas value; pH, blood urea nitrogen (BUN), and partial pressure of carbon dioxide ($pCO_2$) are all blood gas values.

**74. B:** Sodium is the most plentiful electrolyte in serum or plasma.

**75. A:** Both sodium and potassium play a role in maintaining osmotic pressure and acid-base balance; potassium is important in maintaining muscle function and cardiac output. Blood urea nitrogen (BUN) is used to measure renal function.

**76. C:** Human chorionic gonadotropin (HCG) levels are increased during pregnancy; however, HCG may not be present in sufficient levels the first week or 2 after conception, and thus may yield false-negative results. Contaminants such as detergents, protein, hematuria, and bacteria as well as certain medications may invalidate results. Malignant ovarian tumors and other conditions may increase HCG levels.

**77. A:** A long-lasting white foam may indicate renal disease; deeply pigmented yellow foam on yellow-brown or -green urine may indicate the presence of bilirubin or biliverdin, which are associated with hepatitis. Normal urine may range in color from yellow to dark amber. Bacteria and epithelial cells are indicative of a pathological condition only when present in large quantities.

**78. B:** Urinary pH ranges from 5 to 9, with 7 considered neutral. Urine is considered acidic at a pH of less than 7 and alkaline at a pH of greater than 7.

**79. D:** A positive nitrite test in conjunction with a positive leukocyte test is indicative of urinary tract infection (UTI); a urine culture positive for blood or protein is also indicative of UTI. Glucose in the urine may be indicative of diabetes mellitus.

**80. C:** Trough levels are collected when the serum concentration of the drug is at its lowest level, usually just prior to administration of the next dose; peak levels are collected when the serum concentration is highest, usually 30 to 60 minutes after drug administration, and are used to screen for drug intoxication. Neither peak nor trough levels are useful for DNA testing.

**81. B:** The purified protein derivative (PPD) skin test is used to diagnose tuberculosis (TB); the Schick test is used in the diagnosis of diphtheria and the Dick test in the diagnosis of scarlet fever. The histoplasmosis (histo) test is used to test for infection with the organism *Histoplasmosis capsulatum*.

**82. C:** Prior to a fecal occult blood test, patients are prohibited from ingesting foods such as red meat, turnips, horseradish, vitamin C, aspirin, or anti-inflammatory drugs; however, patient are encouraged to eat fruits such as prunes, grapes, or apples and vegetables such as spinach, lettuce, and corn.

**83. B:** Bilirubin is normally present in the blood but not in the urine and is indicative of liver or gallbladder disease or cancer. Albumin is the primary protein found in urine; ketones are end products of fat metabolism and normally present in the urine. Bacteria may be present in the urine in small amounts; only large quantities of bacteria are indicative of pathology.

**84. D:** Cryoglobulin, cryofibrinogen, and cold agglutinin specimens must be kept at or near body temperature; lactic acid, ammonia, and glucagon specimens require chilling.

**85. C:** The transverse plane divides the body into top and bottom halves; the sagittal plane divides the body into unequal right and left halves and the midsagittal plane into equal right and left halves. The frontal plane is parallel to the long axis of the body and at right angles to the midsagittal plane.

**86. D:** The abbreviation q stands for "every"; thus, Q2H means that the drug should be given every 2 hours. BID indicates that the drug should be administered twice a day and PO means given orally (from the Latin *per os*), or by mouth.

**87. A:** Connective tissue is the most common type of tissue found in the body; muscle tissue is essential for movement and epithelial tissue protects the internal and external structures of the body. Nerve tissue consists of cells that send and receive information.

**88. C:** There are a total of 206 bones in the human body.

**89. B:** There are a total of 656 muscles in the body.

**90. C:** The synapse is the area between neurons over which impulses literally jump to transmit messages; dendrites and axons are extensions of the neuron. The myelin sheath covers the axon and increases the speed of a nerve impulse.

**91. B:** The white matter of the brain is composed of the myelin sheath; nonmyelinated axons are not covered by the myelin sheath and are known as the gray matter. Schwann cells are a fatty substance that composes the myelin sheath; synapses are areas between neurons over which impulses jump to transmit messages.

**92. A:** The peripheral nervous system (PNS) is located outside of the central nervous system (CNS) and is composed of the cranial nerves except the optic nerve, the spinal nerves, and the autonomic nervous system. The spinal cord and brain compose the CNS.

**93. D:** Hydrocephalus is an increased volume of cerebrospinal fluid in the brain at birth and is characterized by an enlargement of the infant's head; headache, stiff neck, and fever are symptoms of meningitis, or an inflammation of the meninges of the brain. A shuffling gait, muscular rigidity, and tremor are characteristic of Parkinson disease, and nerve pain is characteristic of neuralgia.

**94. B:** The outermost layer of the skin is known as the epidermis; the second layer, or the dermis, is thicker than the epidermis and is known as the "true skin." The subcutaneous or hypodermal layer lies underneath the dermis.

**95. C:** Hiatal hernia is a condition marked by protrusion of the stomach through a weak area of the diaphragm; gastritis is an acute or chronic inflammation of the stomach lining, and peptic ulcer is erosion of the stomach lining. Gastroesophageal reflux disease (GERD) is a relaxation of the lower sphincter muscle that allows the contents of the stomach to move up the esophagus.

**96. D:** Sweat glands are a type of exocrine gland, which is composed of ducts that carry secretions to the body surface or to organs. The pancreas, pituitary, and thyroid are endocrine glands, or ductless glands that secrete hormones directly into the bloodstream.

**97. B:** Dwarfism is caused by hypofunctioning of the pituitary gland in childhood; Cushing syndrome is caused by hypersecretion of the glucocorticoid hormone and diabetes by reduced secretion of insulin from the pancreas. Parkinson disease is a disorder of the peripheral nervous system.

**98. C:** The throat is also known as the pharynx; the larynx is known as the voice box, and the trachea is known as the windpipe. The epiglottis is a covering of the opening of the larynx that causes food to pass down the esophagus rather than the trachea.

**99. A:** Asthma is caused by obstruction of the airway due to inflammation; bronchitis is caused by inflammation of the bronchial tubes. Hyperventilation is characterized by rapid breathing resulting in a loss of carbon dioxide. Hypoxia is caused by oxygen deficiency.

**100. C:** The major portion of the heart is known as the myocardium; the pericardium is a layer of fibrous tissue that surrounds the heart, and the endocardium covers the inner layer of the heart. The atrium is the receiving chamber of the heart.

**101. A:** The ventricles are the chambers of the heart that pump blood; the right ventricle pumps deoxygenated blood to the lungs and the left oxygenated blood to the rest of the body. The atria are the chambers of the heart that receive blood. The endocardium covers the inner layer of the heart; the septum is the wall of cartilage that separates the four chambers.

**102. C:** The human body has an average of 8 to 10 pints, or 4 to 5 quarts, of blood.

**103. D:** Approximately 92% of plasma is composed of water; the remainder is composed of solutes. Fibrinogen is a plasma protein; electrolytes such as sodium, calcium, and potassium come from food and are found in plasma in smaller amounts.

**104. C:** Aspartate aminotransferase (AST) is typically used to diagnose cardiovascular conditions. Hemoglobin (Hgb), complete blood count (CBC), and erythrocyte sedimentation rate (ESR) are used to diagnose blood diseases such as anemia or leukemia.

**105. B:** The arterial puncture site is typically used for testing arterial blood gases (ABGs); the antecubital veins are used for venipuncture, with the median cubital vein considered the first choice. The veins located in the antecubital fossa are used for venous puncture.

**106. C:** A suprapubic specimen may be collected for infants or small children to ensure that the sample is not contaminated; the clean catch and midstream clean catch methods are used for adults to ensure an uncontaminated specimen. For a regular void specimen, urine is simply collected in a wide-mouth container.

**107. D:** Tests for cerebrospinal fluid (CSF) include total protein, glucose, and chloride; ABO typing is used for paternity testing.

**108. B:** A postprandial (PP) specimen is collected 2 hours after ingestion of a meal; fasting blood sugar (FBS) testing occurs after the patient has fasted 12 hours. Hgb, or hemoglobin, may be collected regardless of meals. HBV stands for hepatitis B virus.

**109. A:** Alcohol, corticosteroids, blood pressure medications, or birth control pills may affect the results of the glucose tolerance test (GTT); aspirin does not affect GTT results.

**110. B:** Activated coagulation time (ACT), prothrombin time (PT), and partial thromboplastin time (PTT) are all used for coagulation monitoring; Hgb, or hemoglobin, is used for the diagnosis of anemia.

**111. C:** The prothrombin time (PT) test may be used in conjunction with partial thromboplastin time (PTT) to assess a patient's total clotting abnormalities; activated coagulation time (ACT) is used to monitor heparin therapy. APPT stands for activated partial thromboplastin time and PP postprandial testing.

**112. B:** As with prothrombin time (PT), activated partial thromboplastin time (APPT) whole blood values differ from plasma values; normal whole blood values range from 93 to 127 seconds and normal plasma values from 24 to 34 seconds.

**113. A:** Blood gas values such as partial pressure of carbon dioxide ($pCO_2$) are typically ordered stat; human chorionic gonadotropin (HCG) is a pregnancy test. The fasting blood sugar (FBS) test is a timed test for which patients must restrict dietary intake for 12 hours. The hemoglobin (Hgb) test is used to diagnose anemia.

**114. C:** Enteric isolation procedures are required for patients with intestinal infections that may be transmitted by ingestion; drainage/secretion isolation is required for burn patients or those with skin infections. AFB (acid-fast-bacilli) isolation is used for patients with tuberculosis.

**115. D:** The Occupational Safety and Health Administration (OSHA) requires that a high-efficiency particulate air (HEPA) respirator be used to protect healthcare workers caring for acid-fast-bacilli (AFB) patients, such as those with infectious tuberculosis; a HEPA respirator is not required for enteric or contact isolation patients or burn patients.

**116. C:** The Occupational Safety and Health Administration (OSHA) requires manufacturers of hazardous chemicals to supply Safety Data Sheets (SDS) for all chemical products; SDS are kept in a laboratory logbook or binder as a reference for lab personnel.

**117. A:** Contaminated needles should never be recapped; the phlebotomist should replace the patient's bed rails after specimen collection and report unusual odors, spills, or dropped items to the nurse.

**118. C:** Environmental conditions such as water, oxygen or lack of oxygen, proper pH, darkness, and proper temperature of 37.5°C or 98.6°F are required for pathogen growth.

**119. B:** Postexposure treatment with hepatitis B immune globulin (HBIG) is effective in preventing HBV; however, no vaccine is available for either HCV or HIV.

**120. C:** Because exposure does not necessarily lead to human immunodeficiency virus (HIV), as well as the potential for serious drug side effects, postexposure treatment is not recommended for all occupational exposures to HIV. No vaccine is available for HIV, and HIV may be transmitted through breast milk. Those exposed to HIV should be tested 6 weeks, 12 weeks, and 6 months after exposure.

**121. B:** The reservoir host is a person, animal, plant, or other organism or substance that acts as the source of transmission of a pathogen; the susceptible host is the person capable of being infected with a pathogen. The chain of infection is the order in which pathogens are transmitted; direct contact is the direct physical transfer of pathogens from a reservoir to a susceptible host.

**122. D:** Personal protective equipment (PPE) such as gloves, mask, and gowns is required when entering the room of a patient under drainage/secretion isolation, such as those with skin infections, AFB isolation, such as those with tuberculosis, or enteric isolation, such as those with intestinal infections that may be transmitted through ingestion; PPE is not required for patients with HIV.

**123. C:** Some chemicals may be activated by water and should not be flushed; the safety data sheets (SDS) should be consulted for detailed information regarding antidotes. Mixing bleach and ammonia creates a gas that may be toxic. Electrical hazards should be moved away from the patient using a broom handle or another object made of glass or wood. Lead aprons and lead-lined gloves are required as a precaution against radioactive hazards.

**124. B:** The accession number, time of test, patient's name and date of birth, and the phlebotomist's initials are required information on specimen tube labels; the physician's signature is required on requisition forms.

**125. D:** Laboratory requisition forms may be transmitted to the laboratory via courier, pneumatic tube system, or in the case of computerized forms, e-mail; verbal laboratory requests may only be given in the outpatient or emergency setting and must be documented on a laboratory requisition form.

**126. B:** When taking calls, the phlebotomist should not wait until the first call is finished before taking another call; ask the first caller for permission to be put on hold, then answer the second call. When the second call is completed, return to the first call. An individual's "personal space," or comfort zone, is based on culture and should be respected. Sign language may be used for both hearing-impaired and non–English-speaking patients.

**127. C:** Negligence is defined as the failure to act, resulting in injury or harm to the patient, and does not require intent to harm. Invasion of privacy is a tort involving use of a patient's name for commercial gain, intrusion into a patient's private life, or disclosure of private information. Abandonment is the premature termination of a professional relationship with a patient without notice or patient consent.

**128. A:** Abandonment, or the premature termination of a professional relationship between a healthcare provider and a patient without notice or patient consent, is an example of an intentional tort; negligence does not require intent. Malpractice is negligence or improper treatment by a health care professional. Chain of custody refers to the procedure for ensuring that specimens have been obtained for the correct patient, have been labeled correctly, and have not been subject to tampering.

**129. C:** Pre- and post- are examples of a prefix, which is added to the beginning of a word to indicate an amount, location, or time; pre- means "before" and post- means "after." A suffix is added to the end of a word and indicates a procedure, condition, or disease, such as "-algia," or pain. An abbreviation is used to shorten a medical term, such as "BID," or twice a day. A root word is the basis of a term and establishes its meaning; for example, "cardi" is a root word meaning heart.

**130. D:** The term caudal means toward the tail, or inferior; cranial means toward the head, or superior. The term medial means toward the midline, and lateral means toward the side of the body.

**131. C:** Glass tubes are preferred for blood alcohol specimens because of the porous nature of plastic tubes; random drug screening may be performed without patient consent, such as in the case of athletes or employees of health care organizations. A split sample may be required for confirmation or parallel testing. A proctor may be required to be present to verify that the specimen was obtained from the correct individual.

**132. A:** Failing to maintain blood pressure at 40 mm Hg may decrease bleeding time; aspirin, ethanol, dextran, or other drugs containing salicylate may prolong bleeding time.

**133. B:** The activated clotting time (ACT) test is used to monitor heparin levels; partial pressure of oxygen ($PO_2$) is an arterial blood gas and ionized calcium an electrolyte. Glucose levels are measured by the 2-hour postprandial (PP) test.

**134. D:** Arsenic, zinc, iron, copper, aluminum, and lead are all examples of trace elements; magnesium is not a trace element.

**135. B:** Measurement of cardiac troponin is useful in the diagnosis of acute myocardial infarction or heart attack; glucose testing is used in diagnosing diabetes. Hematocrit is used for anemia and occult blood for colon cancer screening.

**136. C:** B-type natriuretic peptide (BNP) blood concentrations are measured to detect congestive heart failure; the purified protein derivative (PPD) skin test is used to test for tuberculosis. The Histo and Cocci skin tests are used to test for the fungal infections *Histoplasmosis* and *Coccidioidomycosis*, respectively.

**137. B:** In administering a tuberculosis (TB) skin test, the antigen should be injected just below the skin, not into a vein. Presence of a bleb or wheal indicates that the antigen was injected properly. A TB reaction is measured according to the degree of induration or hardness, not erythema or redness.

**138. C:** A positive reaction to a TB skin test is indicated by induration of 10 mm or greater in diameter; induration between 5 and 9 mm in diameter indicates a doubtful reaction and less than 5 mm in diameter a negative reaction. The degree of redness or erythema is not relevant.

**139. D:** The first step in performing a test for group A streptococci is nitrous acid or enzymatic extraction of the throat swab specimen, followed by latex agglutination or enzyme immunoassay for antigen detection. Specific gravity is measured through urinalysis.

**140. C:** Arterial puncture is primarily performed to evaluate arterial blood gasses (ABGs). Arterial puncture is usually more difficult to perform and more painful than venipuncture; thus, it is not used for routine blood tests.

**141. B:** $PO_2$, or partial pressure of oxygen, is used to measure oxygen levels in the blood; decreased oxygen levels increase the respiration rate and vice versa. $PCO_2$, or partial pressure of carbon dioxide, is used to measure carbon dioxide levels in the blood; increased $CO_2$ levels in the blood increase the respiration rate and vice versa. $HCO_3$ measures the amount of bicarbonate in the blood and is used to evaluate the bicarbonate system in the kidneys. pH measures the acidity or alkalinity of the blood.

**142. D:** Base excess or deficit is used to calculate the nonrespiratory part of acid-base balance and is based on $PCO_2$, $HCO_3$, and hematocrit (Hct) levels; $O_2$ saturation is the percentage of oxygen bound to hemoglobin.

**143. D:** Because the radial artery can be easily compressed over the wrist, it carries a lower risk of hematoma; however, because of its small size, it may be difficult to locate in patients with low cardiac output. If the radial artery is damaged during arterial puncture, the ulnar artery may be used to supply blood to the hand. The radial artery should not be punctured in the absence of collateral circulation.

**144. A:** The femoral artery is located in the groin and is usually used for arterial puncture only in emergency situations or when no other sites are available; arterial specimens may also be obtained from the scalp or from the umbilical arteries in infants. The brachial artery is located in the arm near the insertion of the biceps muscle.

**145. C:** The Allen test is used to assess collateral circulation. In performing the Allen test, both the radial and ulnar arteries should be compressed at the same time to assess the return of blood when pressure is released. The patient should not hyperextend the fingers when opening his or her hand because this may result in decreased blood flow and interfere with results. A positive result is indicated when the hand flushes pink or returns to normal color within 15 seconds.

**146. B:** In infants, the scalp or umbilical artery may be used for arterial puncture. The brachial artery is not used in infants or children because it is more difficult to palpate and lacks collateral circulation. The femoral artery is generally only used in emergency situations or if no other sites are available. The ulnar artery is not used for arterial puncture.

**147. A:** The presence of a bleb or wheal indicates proper injection of a local anesthetic prior to arterial puncture as well as proper injection of the antigen during tuberculosis (TB) testing. Induration or hardness of 10 mm or greater indicates a positive TB reaction. A positive Allen test is indicated by the hand flushing pink or regaining normal coloration within 15 seconds.

**148. C:** The vasovagal response is fainting or loss of consciousness due to a nervous system response to abrupt pain or trauma, and may occur during arterial puncture. A hematoma is the

115

appearance of swelling or a blood mass during or following venipuncture. Myocardial infarction is also known as heart attack.

**149. D:** Serous fluid may be obtained from the peritoneal or abdominal cavity, the pleural cavity surrounding the lungs, or the pericardial cavity surrounding the heart. Cerebrospinal fluid is obtained from the spinal cavity.

**150. B:** The C-urea breath test is used to detect the presence of *Helicobacter pylori*, a form of bacteria causing chronic gastritis and eventually leading to peptic ulcer; the hydrogen breath test is used to assess lactose intolerance. Bone marrow biopsy is used to test for blood disorders and hair samples to detect trace or heavy metals.

# How to Overcome Test Anxiety

Just the thought of taking a test is enough to make most people a little nervous. A test is an important event that can have a long-term impact on your future, so it's important to take it seriously and it's natural to feel anxious about performing well. But just because anxiety is normal, that doesn't mean that it's helpful in test taking, or that you should simply accept it as part of your life. Anxiety can have a variety of effects. These effects can be mild, like making you feel slightly nervous, or severe, like blocking your ability to focus or remember even a simple detail.

If you experience test anxiety—whether severe or mild—it's important to know how to beat it. To discover this, first you need to understand what causes test anxiety.

## Causes of Test Anxiety

While we often think of anxiety as an uncontrollable emotional state, it can actually be caused by simple, practical things. One of the most common causes of test anxiety is that a person does not feel adequately prepared for their test. This feeling can be the result of many different issues such as poor study habits or lack of organization, but the most common culprit is time management. Starting to study too late, failing to organize your study time to cover all of the material, or being distracted while you study will mean that you're not well prepared for the test. This may lead to cramming the night before, which will cause you to be physically and mentally exhausted for the test. Poor time management also contributes to feelings of stress, fear, and hopelessness as you realize you are not well prepared but don't know what to do about it.

Other times, test anxiety is not related to your preparation for the test but comes from unresolved fear. This may be a past failure on a test, or poor performance on tests in general. It may come from comparing yourself to others who seem to be performing better or from the stress of living up to expectations. Anxiety may be driven by fears of the future—how failure on this test would affect your educational and career goals. These fears are often completely irrational, but they can still negatively impact your test performance.

> **Review Video: <u>3 Reasons You Have Test Anxiety</u>**
> Visit mometrix.com/academy and enter code: 428468

## Elements of Test Anxiety

As mentioned earlier, test anxiety is considered to be an emotional state, but it has physical and mental components as well. Sometimes you may not even realize that you are suffering from test anxiety until you notice the physical symptoms. These can include trembling hands, rapid heartbeat, sweating, nausea, and tense muscles. Extreme anxiety may lead to fainting or vomiting. Obviously, any of these symptoms can have a negative impact on testing. It is important to recognize them as soon as they begin to occur so that you can address the problem before it damages your performance.

> **Review Video: 3 Ways to Tell You Have Test Anxiety**
> Visit mometrix.com/academy and enter code: 927847

The mental components of test anxiety include trouble focusing and inability to remember learned information. During a test, your mind is on high alert, which can help you recall information and stay focused for an extended period of time. However, anxiety interferes with your mind's natural processes, causing you to blank out, even on the questions you know well. The strain of testing during anxiety makes it difficult to stay focused, especially on a test that may take several hours. Extreme anxiety can take a huge mental toll, making it difficult not only to recall test information but even to understand the test questions or pull your thoughts together.

> **Review Video: How Test Anxiety Affects Memory**
> Visit mometrix.com/academy and enter code: 609003

## Effects of Test Anxiety

Test anxiety is like a disease—if left untreated, it will get progressively worse. Anxiety leads to poor performance, and this reinforces the feelings of fear and failure, which in turn lead to poor performances on subsequent tests. It can grow from a mild nervousness to a crippling condition. If allowed to progress, test anxiety can have a big impact on your schooling, and consequently on your future.

Test anxiety can spread to other parts of your life. Anxiety on tests can become anxiety in any stressful situation, and blanking on a test can turn into panicking in a job situation. But fortunately, you don't have to let anxiety rule your testing and determine your grades. There are a number of relatively simple steps you can take to move past anxiety and function normally on a test and in the rest of life.

> **Review Video: How Test Anxiety Impacts Your Grades**
> Visit mometrix.com/academy and enter code: 939819

# Physical Steps for Beating Test Anxiety

While test anxiety is a serious problem, the good news is that it can be overcome. It doesn't have to control your ability to think and remember information. While it may take time, you can begin taking steps today to beat anxiety.

Just as your first hint that you may be struggling with anxiety comes from the physical symptoms, the first step to treating it is also physical. Rest is crucial for having a clear, strong mind. If you are tired, it is much easier to give in to anxiety. But if you establish good sleep habits, your body and mind will be ready to perform optimally, without the strain of exhaustion. Additionally, sleeping well helps you to retain information better, so you're more likely to recall the answers when you see the test questions.

Getting good sleep means more than going to bed on time. It's important to allow your brain time to relax. Take study breaks from time to time so it doesn't get overworked, and don't study right before bed. Take time to rest your mind before trying to rest your body, or you may find it difficult to fall asleep.

> **Review Video: The Importance of Sleep for Your Brain**
> Visit mometrix.com/academy and enter code: 319338

Along with sleep, other aspects of physical health are important in preparing for a test. Good nutrition is vital for good brain function. Sugary foods and drinks may give a burst of energy but this burst is followed by a crash, both physically and emotionally. Instead, fuel your body with protein and vitamin-rich foods.

Also, drink plenty of water. Dehydration can lead to headaches and exhaustion, especially if your brain is already under stress from the rigors of the test. Particularly if your test is a long one, drink water during the breaks. And if possible, take an energy-boosting snack to eat between sections.

> **Review Video: How Diet Can Affect your Mood**
> Visit mometrix.com/academy and enter code: 624317

Along with sleep and diet, a third important part of physical health is exercise. Maintaining a steady workout schedule is helpful, but even taking 5-minute study breaks to walk can help get your blood pumping faster and clear your head. Exercise also releases endorphins, which contribute to a positive feeling and can help combat test anxiety.

When you nurture your physical health, you are also contributing to your mental health. If your body is healthy, your mind is much more likely to be healthy as well. So take time to rest, nourish your body with healthy food and water, and get moving as much as possible. Taking these physical steps will make you stronger and more able to take the mental steps necessary to overcome test anxiety.

# Mometrix

## Mental Steps for Beating Test Anxiety

Working on the mental side of test anxiety can be more challenging, but as with the physical side, there are clear steps you can take to overcome it. As mentioned earlier, test anxiety often stems from lack of preparation, so the obvious solution is to prepare for the test. Effective studying may be the most important weapon you have for beating test anxiety, but you can and should employ several other mental tools to combat fear.

First, boost your confidence by reminding yourself of past success—tests or projects that you aced. If you're putting as much effort into preparing for this test as you did for those, there's no reason you should expect to fail here. Work hard to prepare; then trust your preparation.

Second, surround yourself with encouraging people. It can be helpful to find a study group, but be sure that the people you're around will encourage a positive attitude. If you spend time with others who are anxious or cynical, this will only contribute to your own anxiety. Look for others who are motivated to study hard from a desire to succeed, not from a fear of failure.

Third, reward yourself. A test is physically and mentally tiring, even without anxiety, and it can be helpful to have something to look forward to. Plan an activity following the test, regardless of the outcome, such as going to a movie or getting ice cream.

When you are taking the test, if you find yourself beginning to feel anxious, remind yourself that you know the material. Visualize successfully completing the test. Then take a few deep, relaxing breaths and return to it. Work through the questions carefully but with confidence, knowing that you are capable of succeeding.

Developing a healthy mental approach to test taking will also aid in other areas of life. Test anxiety affects more than just the actual test—it can be damaging to your mental health and even contribute to depression. It's important to beat test anxiety before it becomes a problem for more than testing.

> **Review Video: Test Anxiety and Depression**
> Visit mometrix.com/academy and enter code: 904704

# Study Strategy

Being prepared for the test is necessary to combat anxiety, but what does being prepared look like? You may study for hours on end and still not feel prepared. What you need is a strategy for test prep. The next few pages outline our recommended steps to help you plan out and conquer the challenge of preparation.

## STEP 1: SCOPE OUT THE TEST

Learn everything you can about the format (multiple choice, essay, etc.) and what will be on the test. Gather any study materials, course outlines, or sample exams that may be available. Not only will this help you to prepare, but knowing what to expect can help to alleviate test anxiety.

## STEP 2: MAP OUT THE MATERIAL

Look through the textbook or study guide and make note of how many chapters or sections it has. Then divide these over the time you have. For example, if a book has 15 chapters and you have five days to study, you need to cover three chapters each day. Even better, if you have the time, leave an extra day at the end for overall review after you have gone through the material in depth.

If time is limited, you may need to prioritize the material. Look through it and make note of which sections you think you already have a good grasp on, and which need review. While you are studying, skim quickly through the familiar sections and take more time on the challenging parts. Write out your plan so you don't get lost as you go. Having a written plan also helps you feel more in control of the study, so anxiety is less likely to arise from feeling overwhelmed at the amount to cover.

## STEP 3: GATHER YOUR TOOLS

Decide what study method works best for you. Do you prefer to highlight in the book as you study and then go back over the highlighted portions? Or do you type out notes of the important information? Or is it helpful to make flashcards that you can carry with you? Assemble the pens, index cards, highlighters, post-it notes, and any other materials you may need so you won't be distracted by getting up to find things while you study.

If you're having a hard time retaining the information or organizing your notes, experiment with different methods. For example, try color-coding by subject with colored pens, highlighters, or post-it notes. If you learn better by hearing, try recording yourself reading your notes so you can listen while in the car, working out, or simply sitting at your desk. Ask a friend to quiz you from your flashcards, or try teaching someone the material to solidify it in your mind.

## STEP 4: CREATE YOUR ENVIRONMENT

It's important to avoid distractions while you study. This includes both the obvious distractions like visitors and the subtle distractions like an uncomfortable chair (or a too-comfortable couch that makes you want to fall asleep). Set up the best study environment possible: good lighting and a comfortable work area. If background music helps you focus, you may want to turn it on, but otherwise keep the room quiet. If you are using a computer to take notes, be sure you don't have any other windows open, especially applications like social media, games, or anything else that could distract you. Silence your phone and turn off notifications. Be sure to keep water close by so you stay hydrated while you study (but avoid unhealthy drinks and snacks).

Also, take into account the best time of day to study. Are you freshest first thing in the morning? Try to set aside some time then to work through the material. Is your mind clearer in the afternoon or evening? Schedule your study session then. Another method is to study at the same time of day that you will take the test, so that your brain gets used to working on the material at that time and will be ready to focus at test time.

## STEP 5: STUDY!

Once you have done all the study preparation, it's time to settle into the actual studying. Sit down, take a few moments to settle your mind so you can focus, and begin to follow your study plan. Don't give in to distractions or let yourself procrastinate. This is your time to prepare so you'll be ready to fearlessly approach the test. Make the most of the time and stay focused.

Of course, you don't want to burn out. If you study too long you may find that you're not retaining the information very well. Take regular study breaks. For example, taking five minutes out of every hour to walk briskly, breathing deeply and swinging your arms, can help your mind stay fresh.

As you get to the end of each chapter or section, it's a good idea to do a quick review. Remind yourself of what you learned and work on any difficult parts. When you feel that you've mastered the material, move on to the next part. At the end of your study session, briefly skim through your notes again.

But while review is helpful, cramming last minute is NOT. If at all possible, work ahead so that you won't need to fit all your study into the last day. Cramming overloads your brain with more information than it can process and retain, and your tired mind may struggle to recall even previously learned information when it is overwhelmed with last-minute study. Also, the urgent nature of cramming and the stress placed on your brain contribute to anxiety. You'll be more likely to go to the test feeling unprepared and having trouble thinking clearly.

So don't cram, and don't stay up late before the test, even just to review your notes at a leisurely pace. Your brain needs rest more than it needs to go over the information again. In fact, plan to finish your studies by noon or early afternoon the day before the test. Give your brain the rest of the day to relax or focus on other things, and get a good night's sleep. Then you will be fresh for the test and better able to recall what you've studied.

## STEP 6: TAKE A PRACTICE TEST

Many courses offer sample tests, either online or in the study materials. This is an excellent resource to check whether you have mastered the material, as well as to prepare for the test format and environment.

Check the test format ahead of time: the number of questions, the type (multiple choice, free response, etc.), and the time limit. Then create a plan for working through them. For example, if you have 30 minutes to take a 60-question test, your limit is 30 seconds per question. Spend less time on the questions you know well so that you can take more time on the difficult ones.

If you have time to take several practice tests, take the first one open book, with no time limit. Work through the questions at your own pace and make sure you fully understand them. Gradually work up to taking a test under test conditions: sit at a desk with all study materials put away and set a timer. Pace yourself to make sure you finish the test with time to spare and go back to check your answers if you have time.

After each test, check your answers. On the questions you missed, be sure you understand why you missed them. Did you misread the question (tests can use tricky wording)? Did you forget the information? Or was it something you hadn't learned? Go back and study any shaky areas that the practice tests reveal.

Taking these tests not only helps with your grade, but also aids in combating test anxiety. If you're already used to the test conditions, you're less likely to worry about it, and working through tests until you're scoring well gives you a confidence boost. Go through the practice tests until you feel comfortable, and then you can go into the test knowing that you're ready for it.

## Test Tips

On test day, you should be confident, knowing that you've prepared well and are ready to answer the questions. But aside from preparation, there are several test day strategies you can employ to maximize your performance.

First, as stated before, get a good night's sleep the night before the test (and for several nights before that, if possible). Go into the test with a fresh, alert mind rather than staying up late to study.

Try not to change too much about your normal routine on the day of the test. It's important to eat a nutritious breakfast, but if you normally don't eat breakfast at all, consider eating just a protein bar. If you're a coffee drinker, go ahead and have your normal coffee. Just make sure you time it so that the caffeine doesn't wear off right in the middle of your test. Avoid sugary beverages, and drink enough water to stay hydrated but not so much that you need a restroom break 10 minutes into the test. If your test isn't first thing in the morning, consider going for a walk or doing a light workout before the test to get your blood flowing.

Allow yourself enough time to get ready, and leave for the test with plenty of time to spare so you won't have the anxiety of scrambling to arrive in time. Another reason to be early is to select a good seat. It's helpful to sit away from doors and windows, which can be distracting. Find a good seat, get out your supplies, and settle your mind before the test begins.

When the test begins, start by going over the instructions carefully, even if you already know what to expect. Make sure you avoid any careless mistakes by following the directions.

Then begin working through the questions, pacing yourself as you've practiced. If you're not sure on an answer, don't spend too much time on it, and don't let it shake your confidence. Either skip it and come back later, or eliminate as many wrong answers as possible and guess among the remaining ones. Don't dwell on these questions as you continue—put them out of your mind and focus on what lies ahead.

Be sure to read all of the answer choices, even if you're sure the first one is the right answer. Sometimes you'll find a better one if you keep reading. But don't second-guess yourself if you do immediately know the answer. Your gut instinct is usually right. Don't let test anxiety rob you of the information you know.

If you have time at the end of the test (and if the test format allows), go back and review your answers. Be cautious about changing any, since your first instinct tends to be correct, but make sure you didn't misread any of the questions or accidentally mark the wrong answer choice. Look over any you skipped and make an educated guess.

At the end, leave the test feeling confident. You've done your best, so don't waste time worrying about your performance or wishing you could change anything. Instead, celebrate the successful completion of this test. And finally, use this test to learn how to deal with anxiety even better next time.

## Important Qualification

Not all anxiety is created equal. If your test anxiety is causing major issues in your life beyond the classroom or testing center, or if you are experiencing troubling physical symptoms related to your anxiety, it may be a sign of a serious physiological or psychological condition. If this sounds like your situation, we strongly encourage you to seek professional help.

# Thank You

We at Mometrix would like to extend our heartfelt thanks to you, our friend and patron, for allowing us to play a part in your journey. It is a privilege to serve people from all walks of life who are unified in their commitment to building the best future they can for themselves.

The preparation you devote to these important testing milestones may be the most valuable educational opportunity you have for making a real difference in your life. We encourage you to put your heart into it—that feeling of succeeding, overcoming, and yes, conquering will be well worth the hours you've invested.

We want to hear your story, your struggles and your successes, and if you see any opportunities for us to improve our materials so we can help others even more effectively in the future, please share that with us as well. **The team at Mometrix would be absolutely thrilled to hear from you!** So please, send us an email (support@mometrix.com) and let's stay in touch.

> **If you'd like some additional help, check out these other resources we offer for your exam:**
> **http://MometrixFlashcards.com/Phlebotomy**

# Additional Bonus Material

Due to our efforts to try to keep this book to a manageable length, we've created a link that will give you access to all of your additional bonus material.

Please visit https://www.mometrix.com/bonus948/nhaphleb
to access the information.